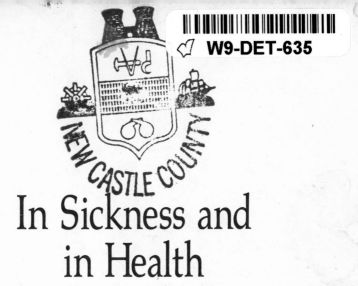

In Sickness and in Health

The Co-dependent Marriage

Mary S. Stuart, R.N., M.S.

Foreword by John Bradshaw

Health Communications, Inc.
Deerfield Beach, Florida

Mary S. Stuart
Denver, Colorado

Quotations from INTIMATE PARTNERS by Maggie Scarf reprinted by permission of Random House, Inc.
Copyright 1987.

Library of Congress Cataloging-in-Publication Data
Stuart, Mary S.
  In sickness and in health.

1. Co-dependence (Psychology) 2. Problem families.
3. Marital psychotherapy. I. Title.
RC569.5.C63S78   1988   362.8′2   88-7217
ISBN 0-932194-73-7

Published by: Health Communications, Inc.
            3201 S.W. 15th Street
            Deerfield Beach, Florida 33442

Cover Design and Illustration by Reta Thomas

DEDICATION

To Hattie Owens (1893-1981)
>   You nurtured me and protected the seeds which
>   have formed my capacity to love. For that I thank
>   you. The pain of missing you is still within me but
>   it is combined with many tender memories of you.

and

To my husband, Larry Keesen
>   You have planted, fertilized, watered, weeded and
>   helped the sun to shine on those seeds . . . my
>   capacity to love. Now they are flowering. Without
>   you, I could not be all of the person I am. I love you.

THANKS TO . . .

My thanks go to many supportive family members and friends for their help and kindness during the writing process.

"John" and "Barbara", who prefer to remain anonymous, and whose marriage serves as the foundation for *In Sickness and in Health* deserve my special gratitude as well as a very special place in my heart. You are each wonderful, loving and inspiring people, uniquely yourselves. Thank you for sharing your lives with me.

And again to my children, Kristin and John, whose love and involvement mean so much to me. You have both made my life immeasurably richer.

Dave Arendt has my gratitude for his help with graphics.

Special thanks to my cousin and friend, Marian Bressel, for her proofreading efforts. And, of course, to my editor and friend, Marie Stilkind, for all of her support and assistance.

John Bradshaw's foreword moved me so much. Thank you, John, for your wonderful contributions.

CONTENTS

TABLES AND FIGURE

FOREWORD

John E. Bradshaw

No subject has any greater urgency than healing co-dependent marriages. Co-dependency is the dis-ease of lost selfhood. Mary S. Stuart, in *Sickness and in Health: The Co-dependent Marriage*, roots co-dependency in the self-rupture of toxic shame. She makes us feel all the barriers to intimacy which are erected in the co-dependent marriage.

My first contact with Mary Stuart was listening to one of her lectures on eating disorders. I learned many important things from Mary, but what impressed me the most was her grounding in healthy shame. Healthy shame makes us human. It gives realistic balance and avoids grandiosity. Mary presents this same balance in *In Sickness and in Health*. We get the benefit of her considerable clinical expertise and we get to laugh at ourselves in the mirror of her self-disclosure. This book is a tremendous contribution to our knowledge about dysfunctional families, marriages and co-dependent behaviors.

Chapters One through Four teach us clearly about co-dependency, both individually and within marriages. They help us identify the origin and expression of this set of problems, and we learn about the many common patterns in co-dependent relationships. Chapter Five offers a concrete way out of the bind of co-dependent entrapment. I found this material especially useful because Mary avoids the rigidity and perfectionistic tone of many writings on recovery from co-dependency.

The importance of this book cannot be overstated. Family dysfunction comes from defective co-dependent marriages. In such families, children are deprived of a model for healthy love and intimacy. Without models, they are forced to repeat their parents' dysfunctions.

In Sickness and in Health offers us ways to stop family dysfunction and multigenerational illness. Please read it!

INTRODUCTION

This book was conceived in the car. My husband and I were driving somewhere and I knew in spite of my self-consciousness that I had to tell him what I had been planning.

"Honey, I'm going to go to an Overeaters Anonymous meeting tomorrow night."

After a moment of silence, he replied, "You don't need that. You don't overeat!"

Let's face it, we're talking heavy duty denial. And when I heaved a sigh of relief and agreed with him we're talking more denial. Why did I weigh so much if not through overeating? A part of me recognized it at the time and I thought to myself, "Other couples must do this too. We keep helping each other maintain ideas about ourselves even though they aren't true at all . . ." But I said nothing.

Larry had a few addictions of his own and since he didn't want me to confront him about his, he was helping me deny my addiction to food. (Both of us have since started the process of recovering from our addictions.) But even the addictions were secondary.

The primary problem was co-dependency and one of its cardinal symptoms: excessive reliance on denial. That conversation made me think about all the couples I had treated over the years and the more I thought, the more related to co-dependency their problems seemed.

Co-dependency is a problem in marriages because the majority of the people in our society are suffering with the symptoms of co-dependency — symptoms like denial, compulsive behavior, depression, anxiety, boundary confusion, problems with control and responsibility plus poor self-esteem.

Okay, so if almost everyone has it, and if our society reinforces it, the institution of marriage must also be afflicted. For lots of reasons.

Successful marriage is a lot harder than it looks. The only training we have for marriage is the attainment of chronological majority. Somehow in the process of growing older, we are supposed to join ourselves with another person and flourish together. We are also to form a healthy and constructive relationship of an intimate nature, and this relationship is to be life-long. A solid and exciting sexual adjustment is also expected, as are healthy and self-actualizing children. All of these expectations combine to explain why nearly one half of the marriages which take place in the United States this year will end in divorce.

In Sickness and in Health was written because of a revealing conversation with my husband. It is a look at marriage from the viewpoint of co-dependency, a disorder which is epidemic in our society. Marriage, which encourages the blurring of boundaries between individuals, and to which we bring the ideals and sicknesses of our families of origin, can mirror the co-dependency of the individual, perhaps better than any other relationship.

Of course, *In Sickness and in Health* will address more than marriage. Any committed relationship, either heterosexual or homosexual, which is entered into with the expectation of permanency, contains the seeds to germinate abundant co-dependency and will therefore be looked at in this volume.

Please forgive me the use of conventional pronouns (he and she, for convenience only) and look for yourself in these pages. Most of us are here.

1
MARRIAGE

A healthy marriage is a rarity in our disordered society. The tasks of marriage are so complex and numerous that it would be difficult for most of us to achieve a healthy marriage even in a less disturbed society. There is no doubt, however, that part of what gets us into trouble with marriage is our expectations.

We are taught that love will conquer all and that falling in love is the answer to problems such as loneliness and addiction. And we marry because we are *"in love"*, not knowing that love can be an addiction as powerful as any narcotic. All this and our capacity to form and maintain relationships must be looked at from their beginnings. Some concept of "normal" is always necessary to understand an "abnormal", and the healthy family is the start of people who are capable of making healthy relationships.

Families Of Origin

Your family of origin is where you grew up. It includes your parents or caretaker and your siblings along with anyone else who lived in the household. You learned about marriage from living in one: your parents'. If your family was a healthy one, your parents had a deep bond of intimacy between them and with you and your siblings.

1

They established consistent spoken and unspoken rules within the family.

Communication in a healthy family is both important and open. This means that if a family member is in need of sharing or conversation, time is made for this. No matter how trivial the subject matter, it is a healthy family's priority to communicate within itself. No one is perfect and sometimes mistakes happen and people don't listen as they should, but for the most part, everyone from the youngest to the oldest member is listened to and respected for their contribution.

Trust is also a priority. Family members are expected to treat each other with kindness and sensitivity to feelings. While life in a healthy family is not routinized, there is predictability. The children know that their needs will be met and the adults can count on each other for support and affection. The family participates in work and play together, and provision is made for the separate interests of the individuals within the family.

If you came from a healthy family, your parents' marriage was your foundation and that of your siblings. Mom and Dad had a close relationship with one another and with their children. The sexual side of their relationship was private but not hidden, and physical affection was often expressed both from one parent to another and from parent to child.

Within the healthy family there is some forum for resolution of conflict. Whether this is a regular family meeting or careful discussion after every disagreement, individuals are encouraged to share their feelings and discuss their opinions.

If your parents were healthy and in a healthy relationship with each other, they taught you to express your feelings by expressing their own feelings and by discussing your feelings with you. They helped you understand yourself and encouraged you, through play and school, to explore new directions and to respect both your limits and your talents.

Your unique learning within a healthy family system did what it was supposed to. It taught you with an open and loving attitude about yourself and other people. And it taught you about marriage by the process of modeling. What you watched for the eighteen years or so you lived within your parents' household was a more effective learning tool than all the television, movies, books, slides and videos ever invented.

Tom remembers his parents with fondness. "They had their problems, and there's no doubt about that. Money was tight much of the time, and my mother developed a form of arthritis at an early age. But they talked to each other about everything, and they talked to all of us and listened when we talked. If I had a problem at school, I was expected to share it with everyone. My parents and my sister discussed it with me and tried to figure out what the options were. The other thing I remember from childhood was play. We often went on picnics and on short drives to the farm communities around our city. Once in a while we took vacations and went fishing or sight-seeing. My mother loved to read and often had a book in her hand. She would read aloud to us if she thought a section was well written or funny. My dad loved to fish and taught both me and my sister how to cast and look for good fishing holes. We were all very affectionate with each other and still are. The house was a warm place to be and my friends all liked to come over and spend time with my parents."

In addition to your parents' marriage, the other pivotal relationship in your early life took place between your parents and yourself. In it you learned what closeness feels like, to trust or not trust, how to separate, and what to expect from others within an intimate relationship.

Your Infancy

The basis of all the close relationships in your life took place when you were a newborn. As far as can be determined, the first experience of the newborn is simply himself. He is unable to distinguish his inner sensations from the outer world. He is completely dependent upon the care of his mother. (Again, the word mother is used to represent the primary caretaker. This could just as easily be the father or someone else altogether.) How well the infant survives depends on the quality of his care, as well as his ability to form an attachment or bond with mother.

Attachment theory (John Bowlby) teaches us that attachment behavior must be encouraged to produce a secure and self-reliant person. If parents provide a secure base and encourage exploration, their child will be able to form constructive attachments throughout his life. Attachment behaviors are those that allow the infant to be closer to the preferred caretaker. This attachment is specific to a single person, enduring through a long period of time, and present in most mammalian species. If caretakers are available and responsive to the infant's needs, and if they provide direction when the infant is floundering, they will provide the nurturing that infants require. They will also set the stage for healthy attachments to others later in life.

To attain normal development, the child must form both a sense of self and relate to others. Soon after birth, and during the first month of life, the infant exists in a sleepy state in which his only world is himself. His entire awareness centers upon his own physiologic processes. Normally, his needs are addressed lovingly by his mother. He is fed when hungry, covered when cold and held when he needs contact.

From the second month of life on, there is the beginning awareness that mother provides for his needs and that she is separate from him, another individual.

Soon the child will smile preferentially at his mother and then will develop growing awareness that there are other people besides himself and mother in the world. As these other people become more apparent, the infant is able to give up some of his fusion with his mother. This is the beginning of his separation from his primary caretaker and the formation of his own special identity.

Just as the movement of limbs and the experience of being held and touched by his mother allows the infant to explore his body boundaries, the emotional connection with his mother allows him to explore his relationships with the rest of the world.

> "When the family environment is satisfactory, the gradual separation of the child from its parents is associated with the development of a coherent and cohesive sense of self."
>
> *Marriage and Mental Illness*

This sense of self is the key to the clear and consistent boundaries that an individual must form if he is to create a healthy, intimate marriage. Without secure individual boundaries, co-dependency is inevitable. In addition, a deficit in his emotional relationship with his mother, or some disturbance in the process of separation will produce long-lasting problems, such as depression, a feeling of emptiness and an inability to trust.

If you learned to love at your mother's breast, you will be able to experience all the richness a life full of relationships can provide. A healthy family of origin provides the foundation for a healthy marriage. A dysfunctional family of origin predisposes to a co-dependent marriage.

Characteristics Of A Healthy Marriage

There are, of course, many varieties of healthy marriage. This is because each marriage is composed of the individuals themselves as well as their particular patterns of intimacy. You will notice that some of the characterisitics of a healthy marriage are the same as those of a healthy family. Essentially, the quality of your parents' marriage set the stage for the quality of your family relationships, which in turn will determine the quality of your own marriage.

The following are the common characteristics of a healthy marriage:

1. Love and a sense of commitment
2. Equal power between partners
3. An interpersonal context
4. Individual autonomy
5. Shared feelings
6. A method for conflict resolution
7. Present orientation
8. Clear boundaries
9. A mutually satisfying sexual relationship
10. A spiritual orientation.

I am fortunate to know two very special people who have been living happily together for many years. They serve as examples of loving human beings in my own life and in the lives of many other people. Their names are John and Barbara. Barbara tells me that, "We do not have a perfect marriage by any means." A fact which I note and respond to by saying that there's no such thing as a perfect marriage because there are no perfect people.

John and Barbara are 74 and 68, respectively, and have been married for 41 years. John is an attractive man with large hazel eyes and silver hair. Barbara is tall and beautiful. Curly grey hair frames her smiling face. You can feel their warmth as soon as you meet them. They had two children, a girl who is now 38 and a boy who would have been 35 had he not died tragically of a brain tumor at the age of 20. They have known each other since John's family moved onto Barbara's street when he was 13 and she was seven. Although they knew each other well, they were not romantically involved until John was 30 and Barbara was 24. At that time John was in the Air Force and World War II was in progress. He was stationed at the base near their home and, because of their proximity, they began dating each other exclusively. Barbara wept when John was transferred to another base much further away.

"I realized what life would be like without John. And I cried when he told me he was being transferred to another base. That was the first time I was aware that I was in love with him," Barbara told me.

They became engaged before he went away, married a year after that and have been together ever since. A good marriage is a wondrous thing to behold. And like an ancient tapestry or an elegant mosaic, it is hard to describe.

Love And A Sense Of Commitment

When you hear the word love, you often think of the popular songs of our era which emphasize pain and suffering and the inability to live without the loved one. That is emphatically *not* what love means within the context of a healthy marriage. This popular-song kind of love contains a remarkable resemblance to addictive drug use, producing highs and lows and being out of control. Healthy love is composed of different feelings altogether.

Healthy love helps both partners feel safe. Their relationship provides them with the feeling that they are secure and that no emotional or physical harm will come to them through their marriage. This is not to say that unpleasant life circumstances, such as illness or failure, will not occur, but the marriage itself will not be the source of these things. Healthy love also provides the feeling that you belong, that you are cared for and that you are important.

In fact, according to Maggie Scarf in *Unfinished Business*,

"Marriage is, when it operates well, a means by which a couple manages to give each other significance. It provides for the adult what the family once provided for the child: a home ground of the soul, an emotional safe shelter. If it works, it is the best sort of mutual support system . . . In the huge life-gamble that is marriage, we put a sense of being 'someone significant' into the hands of another . . . hoping that person will confirm and validate our worth, even as we do his or hers. The bond thus established creates a clearing in an otherwise frightening and impersonal wilderness. Human love attachments, when they flourish, confer a sense that one's existence matters."

Or as John said, "No matter what happens, the love is still there. You go back to first base and it's always love. I mean you really think that much of each other. It's just there."

Along with love there is a sense of commitment to your partner in a healthy marriage. This enables you to feel grounded in the relationship, to pass up opportunities for intimate and sexual relationships with other people. Essentially, a commitment is a pledge, a pledge that you will be there for your spouse no matter what circumstances prevail.

Love also includes the motivation to grow and help assure your partner's growth. Perhaps most important, you and your spouse are friends. You are close and warm and intimate with one another.

John and Barbara express their love for one another with gestures of affection and shared laughter. They accept each other for who they are in spite of differences in their personalities. They share so much together that hearing their reminiscences is special and lovely:

"It was wonderful and we were a very close family."

"And you helped with all the child care, John?"

"Oh, yes . . ." he answered casually, as if this were no big deal. Don't forget, though, that we were talking about a family in the late 1940s, long before active fathering was encouraged.

"John stayed up for the eleven o'clock feeding and I got up for the two o'clock. He helped me with formula and diapers . . ."

John interrupted her, laughing, "Remember those frozen diapers? We had no dryer and they would get board stiff on the clothesline. We'd wash them in the morning and take them off the line in the afternoon."

"He helped me with everything, Mary. Everything. He's been right at my side all these years."

Equal Power

Equal power in a relationship means that both partners have a say in decisions which affect their lives. For many generations, women were expected to give themselves into marriage without the same kind of commitment from their partners. Men were allowed control over such things as place of residence, money and how it was spent and child-rearing. In many parts of the world they were also allowed extramarital sexual liaisons prohibited for women.

In a relationship based on equal power, both partners have equal responsibility and input into decisions about their lives. Both partners are expected to be faithful. Essentially, a relationship in which there is equal power is a feminist relationship because there is no inequality based on gender.

John and Barbara explored the whole issue of power. Money is often a symbol of how power is handled in a marriage. John and Barbara share the mechanics of handling money much as they do other things in their lives.

"John had his own money and I never had any before we were married. But I learned in the first few months that someone had to be responsible for the bills."

"We started out with an envelope system and I was completely satisfied with Barbara handling all of the finances."

"And I won't balance the checkbook," Barbara told me with a smile. "So John balances the checkbook and I pay every bill the day we get it. We've never been in debt but sometimes I've had to say I've over-spent. Then we'd take out extra money from savings. In all these years, he has never made an unkind remark about money . . ."

There are no power problems in a healthy relationship because power is shared, not competed over. Some matters are individual decisions and some are couple decisions but the differences are usually clear in a healthy marriage. In addition, in a healthy marriage "winning means winning with and not against. In relationships there is never really one winner and one loser; two people either win or lose together." (Maggie Scarf)

John and Barbara seem to have evolved a naturally equal relationship in which the power is shared. They attribute this to their similar backgrounds, their long experience of each other and their age at the time of their marriage. In addition, their love and good intentions toward one another are clearly part of their shared power. No one is trying to win.

Intimacy is impossible when there are large power differences. In fact, "only in situations of equal overt power can there be intimacy — the experience of being open, vulnerable and able to share one's innermost feelings and thoughts." (W. Beavers) As you can see, equal power allows intimacy and without intimacy, marriage is an empty experience at best.

Interpersonal Context

An interpersonal context is a social system. At the beginning of a relationship the couple usually spends a great deal of time alone with each other in order to establish a bond. When this bond becomes more secure, the couple finds it needs more social interaction. John and Barbara speak fondly of many friends over the years, one of whom taught them a valuable lesson after their own son's death.

"These friends of ours have a son who is deficient. He's not really retarded, but he is deficient. He's a dear son to them. We have watched her struggle all these years with that. She'd go to every one of his teachers explaining why Jimmy couldn't do this or understand that. And Jimmy made a friend of everyone. They all helped him and he graduated from high school. But the hours she spent at school and helping him with his work! And she said to me one day when I was grieving, 'Just remember, you had Steven whole and beautiful for 20 years . . .' That's when I realized that I should be grateful, not angry."

Friends are made, both individually and as a couple. And the marital relationship supports friendship. Social activities are important to the healthy couple, both to meet needs not met within the relationship and for fun. No one can meet all the needs of their spouse, and a social context allows other needs to be met. A healthy couple is not isolated.

If family members live nearby, they, too, fill an important role in the lives of the couple. John and Barbara allude repeatedly with warmth to their relationships with many members of their families. This speaks, of course, to the resolution of the old issues and problems of the family of origin.

Individual Autonomy

Autonomy can be defined as freedom and a sense of complete-ness. If you are autonomous, you are secure in your own worth and unafraid of your individual identity. A healthy marriage supports the individual in his or her personal choices and celebrates each partner's identity.

John is obviously proud of Barbara's skill as a teacher of children who are slow learners. "The kids who are doing well today due to what she did with them in the classroom then . . ." he said. Underneath his words were the unspoken understanding of Barbara's unique talents and accomplishments. This understanding has been expressed in a lifetime of shared work and play and in the one recurring problem that frustrates both partners: Barbara's life-long problem with self-esteem.

John and Barbara recognize each other's differences and strengths and support independence within one another. They have shared activities as well as separate ones, spend time together but also apart. Their autonomy gives them each more to share with the other.

Shared Feelings

Sharing feelings requires both consistent interest in one another and the ability to identify and verbalize different feeling states. No one can identify every feeling easily, but intimate partners can help each other by providing support and sharing how they feel in the same situation.

Active listening is the other side of sharing, for who can share without feeling listened to and attended? Caring and attention go hand in hand, and people don't really share unless they feel cared for. "Since true listening is love in action, nowhere is it more appropriate than in marriage." (Scott Peck)

Because John was recovering from a broken hip, one incident came up in which he shared his feelings with Barbara. "He has only once become angry about this broken hip and it gives me strength to watch how well he can cope with it. He said, 'Lying in bed you feel fine and then you get up and there's that damn hip again.' One day he got angry and bitter about it and he came to me. I said, 'You have a right to be mad . . . it's okay'."

Barbara and John share their tender and positive feelings, as well as their heartfelt and honest laughter. Sharing helps bridge the gap between people. We are not all the same. We are all unique but sharing and listening allow us to find our common ground together. And in sharing negative feelings, one partner can gain helpful support and feedback from the other.

Conflict Resolution

Marriages must have constructive means to resolve the conflicts which inevitably occur in performing the major tasks of living life together. Many difficult and complex jobs are encountered in marriage. Two people, each with their own values and background, are bound to clash over such issues as child-rearing, aging parents, illness and financial management. Without some method of compromise, some bending of wills, every marriage would be mired in continuous resentment.

The best marriages resolve conflict by first determining the needs of each partner and the needs of the couple. Then with the expression of feelings and in a loving and supportive manner, the goals of the couple are defined. Hopefully, both points of view are considered in decision-making and an equitable solution to most problems can be arrived at. Sometimes, one person's needs will take precedence over the other's, but decisions should not always favor the same partner.

Finally, there are some resolutions which can be made within a marriage.

"We never go to bed mad at each other," John told me.

"We always talk about it, but I may still say that I'm right . . . And it's not always easy to resolve things with John, because he won't blow up and yell . . ."

Even with their differences in personal style, there is acceptance between John and Barbara, and a consistent attempt from each of them to find solutions to their problems. There is also a mutual unwillingness to let problems separate or drive a wedge between them. They agree to disagree, rather than spend a night angry with one another.

Present Orientation

A present orientation occurs on two levels: past marital issues and conflicts should stay in the past as should past family of origin issues. Conflicts which were resolved in the past do not need to be continuously resurrected. And problems you bring from your family of origin should not be attributed to your marital relationship.

Healthy people function fully in the now and healthy marriages do the same. In spite of our focus on the history of John and Barbara's marriage, they talked clearly about their families of origin but left them in the past. Problems which remain from those families are recognized as being a result of past issues and the marriage is not blamed for them.

Barbara's long-standing difficulties with self-esteem began in a perfectionistic and praise-withholding family, but she makes a clear distinction between the way she was treated in her family and the way John treats her. She has trouble accepting praise from anyone, but she knows John does praise her and that the problem cannot be attributed to their marriage. John is concerned because of the pain Barbara lives with as a result of her poor self-esteem. While he gives her positive feedback and lots of support, he doesn't take responsibility for her problem.

Clear Boundaries

The word boundary when used in this context describes the sense of self, where I end and you begin. We begin to develop our boundaries early in life and . . .

> "By the end of the first year we know that this is my arm, my foot, my head, my tongue, my eyes and even my viewpoint, my voice, my thoughts, my stomachache and my feelings. We know our size and our physical limits. These limits are our boundaries. The knowledge of these limits inside our minds is what is meant by ego boundaries. The development of ego boundaries is a process that continues through childhood into adolescence and even into adulthood, but the boundaries established later are more psychic than physical."
>
> *Scott Peck*

Without boundaries there is no stable sense of self since we are always merging into someone else. In a healthy marriage the sense of self is well established in both partners and both know where they begin and end and whose feelings belong to whom.

Nowhere is it more difficult to establish clear boundaries than with a sick child. When Steven was having treatment for his brain tumor, he insisted upon going back to school, trying to live a normal life in spite of the side effects from chemotherapy. Barbara spoke for both herself and for John when she told me, "It destroyed us when he went back to school, but he wanted to. And it was his life and he had to do what he wanted with the rest of it . . ."

John and Barbara have a lot in common, but they are different, too. Each is aware of their differences and each is clear about who is who.

A Mutually Satisfying Sexual Relationship

Mature adults require sexual contact with one another as a kind of booster to intimacy. Sexual interchange leads to orgasm which allows a physical release of sexual tension and a feeling of emotional closeness. This helps people to transcend the difficulties even close human beings have in day-to-day life together.

Sexual athletics are not necessary, and there is no normal number of sexual encounters in a given period of time for everyone. As long as both partners are satisfied with the number and kind of exchanges and have most of their sexual needs met most of the time, their sexual relationship is adequate. Healthy marriages do not rely on any given kind of sexual exchange. Although there are favorite positions and techniques, a wide range of activities are available to the couple; activities which are neither offensive nor hurtful to either partner.

In Barbara's and John's marriage, sexuality is an ongoing and mutually comforting and delightful experience in spite of recent medical problems which have forced them to discontinue having sexual intercourse. A minor surgical procedure would allow Barbara to have intercourse again, but although she wants to have it done, John does not want her to go through it. He indicates that continued sexual play and the affection they share is very satisfying for him. And that the most important thing is just being together.

A Spiritual Orientation

Spirituality can be different from organized religion. While some of us can be at our spiritual best in church or temple, some of us prefer a solitary walk in the forest or private meditation. All of these things are spiritual and none are better than others. Spiritual expression is individual and there are no "right" or "wrong" ways to get in touch with your own.

According to Father Leo Booth in *Spirituality and Recovery*, ". . . Spirituality is in being real.

Spirituality reflects the Power that God
    has given every one of us.
Spirituality stops your waiting for a
    miracle, looking for a miracle,
        asking for a miracle.
Spirituality reminds you that *you are the*
    miracle . . ."

In John's and Barbara's lives, spirituality plays a central role. Both are active and committed to their Protestant church and they see their relationship with God as a most important part of their lives.

In fact, they told me, "We live each day in the care of the Lord."

I am grateful to have had a glimpse into a marriage like this and for my ongoing relationship with John and Barbara. Their marriage feels like an ideal to strive for. Unfortunately, many marriages have nothing in common with Barbara's and John's and instead are difficult, even treacherous.

2
PERSISTENT MARITAL ISSUES

There are several issues which surface throughout the life of a marriage, issues with which all couples grapple at one time or another. Because you will be reading about them as they relate to co-dependency, they deserve, it seems to me, a detailed look.

Closeness And Distance

Ideally, of course, each marital partner wants the same amount of closeness as well as like amounts of closeness all the time. But ideals are not reality and the truth is that most of us, depending where we are emotionally at any given time, have varying needs for closeness at varying times in our lives. This is why functional marriages move back and forth, depending on the needs of the individuals, along the continuum of closeness and distance.

For example, if your spouse is involved with a demanding professional project lasting for several days, he or she will probably require more emotional distance from you because of the energy being devoted to the project. With luck, you will be able to tolerate this distance, perhaps even engage in activities of your own.

It is not that your connection breaks but rather, like a piece of elastic, it stretches. What if you are in the midst of a major transition yourself, or a loss? In this case, your partner must be able (for the most part) to return to you, get closer, preserve the reassurance your intimacy can provide. Marriage is dynamic, and both the needs of each individual and the needs of the couple must be met. One of the tasks of marriage is to build a bond which connects you with your spouse despite conflicts and needs at variance with each other. It is not just that you are "in love" but that you are concerned, caring and loving.

Problems will surface when one partner needs, rigidly and consistently, more distance or closeness than the other. Several authors have referred to this type of problem as the pursuer-distancer conflict. It is certainly a conflict as well as a recurring theme within a relationship; a script in which each partner plays a proscribed and consistent part.

According to Maggie Scarf,

> "The pursuer has split off, denied and dissociated any self of her own; autonomy needs are perceived as selfish and bad and can be recognized only as they exist in the mate. The distancer obliges by needing ever-greater areas of individual turf — and the more she chases after him for closeness, the greater is his need for space. Intimacy is . . . something which could swallow a person alive . . . (and he) cannot experience the wish for emotional communion on his own, for it would make him feel so much at risk, so vulnerable to rejection and abandonment."

As Maggie Scarf further points out, the rule here is that the pursuer continues to chase the distancer and that he continues to distance. They never catch up with one another and, therefore, they protect each other from their fears of closeness.

Guerin *et al* discuss pursuit and distance as part of an individual's style which is determined both by family of origin and by the qualities of the marriage. They enumerate the characteristics of the pursuer and distancer.

Table 2.1. Pursuer-Distancer Characteristics

PURSUER	DISTANCER
Wants relationship time	Alone time or activities
Expresses emotions/thoughts	Avoids feelings
Open boundaries	Closed boundaries
Full speed or dead halt	Deliberate pace

Pursuit and distancing in a marriage provide the couple with a stability of sorts until there is stress on the relationship. Then the patterns provide an arena of conflict and a recognizable pattern.

Guerin *et al* have formulated the following table to illustrate "The Interactional Sequence" between pursuers and distancers.

Table 2.2. Interactional Sequence

	EMOTIONAL PURSUER	EMOTIONAL DISTANCER
Step 1:	Moves toward the distancer	Moves away, usually toward objects
Step 2:	Pursues the distancer intensely	Distances more intensely
Step 3:	Tires of pursuit, moves away from the distancer in reactive distance	Moves tentatively toward the pursuer, then away
Step 4:	Attacks the distancer, defending self	Attacks the pursuer, defending self
Step 5:	Remains at fixed distance, not moving toward distancer	Remains at fixed distance, not moving toward pursuer

As you can see, this predictable interactional sequence moves the pursuer closer to the distancer during times of conflict or stress. The distancer requires more space, so he moves away, which distresses the pursuer even more. If this happens occasionally, the couple can usually restore their close connection after the acute stress has been resolved.

> "If the stress and anxiety remain high, however, and this pattern recycles more and more rapidly, the disappointment, anger and hurt begin to accumulate.
> Eventually the emotional pursuer tires of moving forward for connection with only limited success, feels a loss of self-respect and begins to withdraw. The anger and resentment intensify and build toward bitterness."
>
> Guerin *et al*

Essentially, escalation of the conflict creates a stalemate which meets the needs of neither partner.

There are closeness/distance conflicts at times in every marriage. If the couple communicates and neither is locked into fixed behaviors, these are resolved with time and discussion. When closeness/distance conflicts are not resolved, they deteriorate into chronic tension and unresolved hurt and can destroy marriages.

Intimacy And Individuality

There is no way to overstate this: A major issue in every marriage is how to maintain your individual identity and still be intimate with your spouse. This, of course, is related to the closeness/distance issue, but it is also separate from it. Intimacy is that knowledge of one another, that sharing and openness which creates the cornerstone for the marriage, the foundation for the lifetime partnership. Without it, marriage is like an empty, unstable and unfinished house.

> "Intimacy describes a special quality of emotional closeness between two people. It is an affectionate bond, the strands of which are composed of mutual caring, responsibility, trust, open communication of feelings and

sensations, as well as the non-defended interchange of information about significant emotional events . . . activities are more enjoyable and life is richer and more colorful when shared with an intimate partner . . . without intimate relationships, we tend to get lonely and become depressed. The availability of intimate relationships is an important determinant of how well we master life's crises."

H.S. Kaplan

Clear personal boundaries are a precondition for healthy intimacy. Or according to Maggie Scarf, "(the) . . . most pervasive of marital problems (is) distinguishing which feelings, wishes, thoughts, etc., are within the self and which are within the intimate partner. The dilemma has to do with the drawing of personal boundaries . . ."

Boundaries are what separate the limits of your self from the limits of other people. And intimacy requires clear boundaries so that we can be close with one another without losing our unique identities.

When boundaries aren't clear, true intimacy is impossible because people fuse. Fusion occurs when people don't feel safe within their own identities and are constantly trying to become what they think their spouses want or what they think they "should" be. Eventually the only conclusion to this state of affairs is anger and resentment, continued loneliness and a feeling of emptiness and despair.

Boundary disturbance can show up in both the extreme of insulating and barricading against intrusion or investing so much in the outside world that the boundary is effectively destroyed. Figure 2.1 below symbolically describes these.

W.R. Beavers isolates several fears which he calls boundary disturbance themes. These include:

- the fear of going berserk and destroying others
- the fear of sexual misconduct
- the fear of the persons or things projected on

- the fear of being swallowed
- a strange sense of emptiness.

Figure 2.1. Boundaries In Marriage

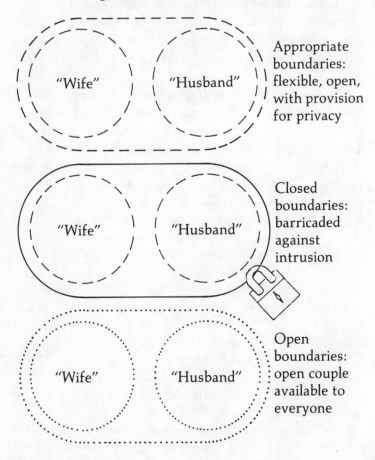

Appropriate boundaries: flexible, open, with provision for privacy

Closed boundaries: barricaded against intrusion

Open boundaries: open couple available to everyone

He further states that, "To live a satisfying life requires a close relationship where one is known and accepted. Unfortunately, these are often avoided for fear of being swallowed, engulfed, taken over, of becoming nobody. Emotional and sometimes physical distance can be experienced as the only way to maintain the tenuous existence of the self."

Projective Identification

Another important concept is projective identification. This concept relates to boundaries and intimacy and appears in virtually all professional discussions of marriage. It is a common, if unconscious mechanism in intimate relationships. In projective identification we attribute characteristics to our spouse which we repudiate within ourselves.

A series of excellent examples of projective identification appear in Maggie Scarf's *Intimate Partners.*

> "According to John Zinner and Roger Shapiro, projective identification is a defensive activity of the ego which serves to modify a person's perceptions of his intimate partner while — in a reciprocal fashion — altering his own image of himself. The individual who is seething with unconscious hostility can, for instance, remain utterly out of contact with those feelings and experience himself as completely without anger — as long as he is assisted by a collusive, obliging mate who will act out his anger for him.
>
> "In other words, it is not enough to have one person project his repudiated and disavowed qualities and emotions — such as his angry feelings — onto the other. The spouse must then conform to the projection, by behaving or feeling in just the ways that she or he is supposed to! It is, in short, a deal; if there is to be a game, two players have to agree, albeit unconsciously, to play it."

When projective identification is used within a marriage, neither partner can be who they truly are. Spouses don't even know one another, but instead relate as if they and their spouses are who they want them to be. Intimacy is completely blocked.

The basis for this behavior is the ambivalence, or uncertainty, about intimacy. It is the combined fear of and desire for closeness and intimacy with which many people are left after experiencing their own parents' ambivalent marriage.

Projective identification is also related to one's inability to tolerate certain emotions. Some of us have had bad experiences with anger: abuse or out-of-control expressions of rage. Because this is so scary, we might want to disavow our own angry feelings. That is when we project them onto our marital partner.

Or as W.R. Beavers states:

> "A frequent shared projective mechanism is the unholy bargain that goes as follows: 'I have ambivalence and you have ambivalence that is painful to resolve. You take the top half of mine and I'll take the bottom half of yours and we will fight like hell. That will feel better than the war inside.' "

Marital Poisons

Poisons kill and marital poisons kill communication. Issues which predictably disrupt marital interaction include money, sex, death and substance abuse. These sometimes serve as a means around which to organize marital conflict; all disagreements can be used to incorporate endless argument about them. All are inter-related: money and sex are often metaphors for power within the relationship and are used to express control.

Power and control can become central issues in a marriage, especially when one or both partners come from controlling parents. A person with this kind of history learns that power is love and that controlling behavior is usual and acceptable. Controlling behaviors run the gamut from constant criticism to humiliation in front of others to threats of physical harm. Often the issues of power and control show up as conflicts about sex or money.

Sexual conflicts of this nature should be suspected when one partner constantly complains about the amount, kind, timing of sex. This is done in an accusa-tory manner and the other spouse defends herself. (The woman is usually, but not always, in this role: "Not tonight, dear. I have a headache.") Accusations and defense about the kind of (or lack of) sex continue and the problem recycles as an endless unresolvable conflict.

Usually this kind of scenario is a result of the real problems remaining unaddressed while each individual struggles continuously with the symptoms. In this type of struggle, the fears are usually about being vulnerable and dependent. They cannot be resolved as long as sex remains the focus.

Fights about money are the other big masquerade for power-struggling. When the fights about money are continuous, the real question is: "Who's in charge?"

According to Jurg Willi,

"Marital power struggles which lead to marriage therapy frequently prove to be resistant to treatment. Therapy sessions become battle sessions . . . The partners often behave like two children in a nursery school. Each accuses the other . . . and presents their point of view with hair-splitting exactness, trying to prove that they have a better case than their partner. Their arguments are carefully based on facts, but differ in emphasis and interpretation. As soon as one feels threatened by the evidence of the other, they introduce new incidents which open up the offensive . . . They attack each other incessantly because they fear that the slightest evidence of weakness will mark them . . . both partners want in reality to avoid separation and to continue the struggle for power."

Death can bring up money issues by raising the specter of inheritance, medical bills and the like; it also acts to release the expression of strong emotions like grief, mourning, anger and ambivalence. And, of course, it can be the resolution or the resurrection of old family of origin issues which may never have been resolved. Sometimes a family death is the catalyst for a couple seeking help.

Substance abuse, most commonly alcohol abuse, is another poison in a relationship. Substance abuse or any other kind of addiction shuts down communication. This kind of problem appears commonly in the co-dependent marriage.

Positions

There are many possibilities for positions within a marriage; these have to do with the roles couples play with one another. In dysfunctional marriages these positions have in common the lack of true intimacy, little trust and closeness and poor individual and couple growth.

> "What is fought out between the mates is . . . the problem neither one of them has been able to address internally — the problem of how to be a distinct and separate individual while remaining emotionally attached to another human being."
>
> *Scarf*

The enmeshed marital position keeps the couple tangled up with one another so that it is never clear who's acting how and for what. Often marriages which are enmeshed are full of chaos, problems and rage. Instead of each individual taking responsibility for their own behavior, they blame one another.

The detached marital position keeps people emotionally separated from one another. They share little and seem to have nothing in common except for children and a shared residence. The detached marriage reminds me of two children playing separate games but sitting next to each other with little or no communication between them. They simply have different agendas.

The controlling marital position includes constant power-struggling and scorekeeping to see who is "winning". Instead of partners, these people are adversaries locked in combat. Sometimes the fighting is overt and sometimes it is more subtle but the outcome is usually predicated on a "winner" and a "loser".

In contrast, the functional or healthy marriage provides an intimate, loving and trusting relationship so that each partner may grow, together and separately. Each spouse is emotionally available to the other. Neither has fears about making "I" or "I feel" statements. Each can be all of themselves.

3
CO-DEPENDENCY

The word co-dependency refers to a set of symptoms which result from growing up in a dysfunctional family. It is estimated that 80% to 90% of us have some of the symptoms of co-dependency. One author, A.W. Schaef, believes that our entire society encourages co-dependency.

Because the dysfunctional family produces the co-dependent individual, we need to look closely at its characteristics. Keep in mind the multi-generational nature of dysfunctional families. Co-dependent individuals from dysfunctional families make co-dependent marriages, and these co-dependent marriages serve as the cornerstone for yet another generation of dysfunctional families. These produce still more co-dependent individuals.

The Dysfunctional Family

One of the ways a family is dysfunctional is when one or more family members is addicted to alcohol or drugs. In fact, if family members are locked into any compulsive behavior (eating, dieting, working, gambling, compulsive sexual behavior), the family becomes dysfunctional. Essentially, if an adult member of a family is engaged in compulsive or addictive behavior, his or her role as parent and spouse is sacrificed to his or her driven-ness and preoccupation with a substance or compulsive activity of choice. This prevents him or her from devoting energy to the family.

The Johnsons brought their daughter after their family doctor referred her to me for the treatment of an eating disorder. Jody was 13 years old, five feet tall, and weighed 150 pounds. She spent most of her time when not in school alone in the house. Her grades had fallen, her activities had declined, and she was barely passing her classes in seventh grade. She appeared sad and angry for reasons which quickly became apparent. The Johnsons were trying to succeed at a business. They had opened a restaurant about two years prior to my initial interview with Jody and were rarely home. Jody had never been a slender child, but since the restaurant opened, she had gone from a high average weight to an obese weight. It didn't take much prodding to get Jody to talk about her loneliness:

"Jody, can you tell me what's going on with you these days?"

"Not much, really."

"Something is making you feel pretty empty so that you have to eat so much."

"I'm always by myself. We used to have a dog, but he died when I was eight. And I used to have a friend next door, but she moved to Wisconsin. My mom and dad are never home anymore."

"Not even at night?"

"No. I go to bed by myself. They call on the phone though. And I see them before I go to school in the morning. They're still in bed."

"That sounds lonely."

"It is."

Both Johnsons were compulsive workers, and they had really not noticed how depressed Jody had become because they were caught up in their business. Jody covered her sadness with food.

After a few family sessions, the Johnsons began to trade days — they alternated spending time at their restaurant with spending time at home. On weekends Jody joined them at the restaurant. A new puppy was adopted from the Humane Society. Within a few months Jody was losing weight and improving her grades.

Compulsive and addictive families are not the only types which produce co-dependency in their members. Any family which is repressive is also dysfunctional. If your family discouraged you from expressing your feelings, you are probably co-dependent.

Many dysfunctional families force their members into rigid roles. One member plays hero and can do no wrong. One member plays victim and is always helpless to affect his or her circumstances. One might withdraw and become lost; one might play comedian and joke all the time. These roles serve to keep the family in its dysfunctional state, but do not allow the individual family member to attain maximum emotional and spiritual growth.

If there is inappropriate sexual behavior between family members whether it is actual incest or covert seductive behavior, the family is dysfunctional. Because a family is a system in which each part affects the whole, any incestuous relationship affects everyone. Dysfunctional families have lots of secrets, both from each other and from the community in which they live. Incest, of course, is one of the most destructive.

Dysfunctional families may engage in constant arguing which produces ever present tension within the family.

Jayne, the adult child of a dysfunctional family, vividly remembers lying in her bed at night listening to her parents shout at one another.

"At first I used to pray they wouldn't get divorced. But after a while I just wanted them to stop fighting. They never did."

Sometimes children are drawn into the parental war to be used as scapegoats and/or distractions. This is emotionally abusive to the child. Physical abuse also occurs in this type of family because one or both parents often grew up in a violent home.

Enmeshment is another characteristic of the dysfunctional family. *Enmeshment* means that people are not free to take distance in their relationships with other family members, that they are all tangled up together. No true emancipation can take place because people are expected to fulfill their old rigid and static roles within the family.

My patient, Amanda, was especially articulate about this conflict. "I moved 2,000 miles away from them, but every time we have a phone conversation I'm in the same old role of bad child. I'm 36 years old and my father can still reduce me to tears with his sarcasm and verbal abuse. My mother still calls me and screams when she's angry at my father. And I can't seem to stop them from doing it." You're never allowed to leave a dysfunctional family.

The dysfunctional family is isolated both from its own members and from the community. People within the family do not share their thoughts and feelings and the family keeps to itself, confiding in no one.

Everyone in a dysfunctional family is expected to be perfect or at least to look perfect. Family members are not taught they can learn from their mistakes, but rather that they must not make them or if they do, they must tell no one.

In summary, compulsive and addictive behaviors, repression, rigid roles, secrets, inappropriate sexual behaviors, enmeshment, isolation, perfectionism, tension and anxiety are the major traits of the dysfunctional family. As you have no doubt observed, these are polar opposites of the traits of the healthy family system.

Sometimes people in dysfunctional families are abused, either physically or emotionally. It has been my experience that this is minimized and although you might have been constantly criticized or called names, or often slapped or even punched, your tendency is to deny the serious nature of this. These types of abuse cause permanent scars which unless they are resolved, can paralyze you.

Many authors call dysfunctional family systems "shame-bound" because shame has such a large influence in family interactions.

Fossum and Mason state the rules of the dysfunctional family, which they call the "shame-bound system". The eight rules are:

1. **Control.** Be in control of all behavior and interactions.
2. **Perfection.** Always be 'right'. Do the 'right' thing.
3. **Blame.** If something doesn't happen as you planned, blame someone (self or other).
4. **Denial.** Deny feelings, especially the negative or vulnerable ones like anxiety, fear, loneliness, grief, rejection, need.
5. **Unreliability.** Don't expect reliability or constancy in relationships. Watch for the unpredictable.
6. **Incompleteness.** Don't bring transactions to completion or resolution.
7. **No talk.** Don't talk openly and directly about shameful, abusive or compulsive behavior.
8. **Disqualification.** When disrespectful, shameful, abusive or compulsive behavior occurs, disqualify it, deny it or disguise it.

The Role Of Shame

Shame is a very important part of the picture of both co-dependency and the dysfunctional family. The dysfunctional family produces a sense of shame in its members. Shame is the feeling that you have been exposed to public view in all of your badness. It is a pervasive sense of inadequacy and hopelessness about yourself. It's not that you have done something bad (guilt), but that you *are* bad.

"Shame is an inner sense of being completely diminished or insufficient as a person. It is the self judging the self. A moment of shame may be humiliation so painful or an indignity so profound that one feels one has been robbed of his or her dignity or exposed as basically inadequate, bad, or worthy of rejection. A pervasive sense of shame is the ongoing premise that one is fundamentally bad, inadequate, defective, unworthy, or not fully valid as a human being." "The roots of shame are in abuse, personal violations, seductions and assaults where one's sense of self had been trampled, one's boundaries defiled."

Fossum and Mason

Long before the focus on dysfunctional families, Erik Erikson, a classically trained analyst, formulated a theory about the developmental stages we all must traverse to attain maturity. One of his early stages includes shame.

"From the sense of inner goodness emanates autonomy and pride; from the sense of badness emanates doubt and shame . . . Shame is early expressed in an impulse to bury one's face or sink, right then and there, into the ground. But this, I think, is essentially rage turned against the self. He who is ashamed would like to force the world not to look at him, not to notice his exposure . . . destroy the eyes of the world. Instead he must wish for his own invisibility. Too much shaming does not result in a sense of propriety but in a secret determination to try to get away with things when unseen . . . there is a limit to a child's and an adult's endurance in the face of demands which force him to consider himself, his body, his needs and his wishes evil and dirty . . ."

Erikson

Shame even has physical manifestations such as blushing and downcast eyes. When you are ashamed, your actions are designed to make yourself smaller, less visible. You will sink into your chair, hang your head and hunch over.

Shame is the province of both the family and the individual. The family hands it down with rigid rules, inability to talk about feelings, abuse and perfectionism; the individual lives it out in co-dependency. Shame is the hallmark and foundation of dysfunctional family systems and individual and marital co-dependency. Unless treated, it is passed from generation to generation.

The Anatomy Of Co-dependency

Each characteristic of co-dependency relates to both individuals and relationships. A co-dependent relationship takes place between two co-dependent individuals, and individual characteristics can then be seen as part of the relationship itself.

When a person or relationship is co-dependent, several of the following symptoms are present:

- excessive reliance on denial
- compulsive behaviors and addictions
- poor self-esteem
- boundary and responsibility problems
- problems with intimacy
- depression and anxiety
- stress-related illnesses.

Excessive Reliance On Denial

Denial is a defense mechanism which prevents difficult and painful feelings, thoughts, impulses and knowledge from being perceived by the conscious mind. Essentially, we refuse to admit to ourselves that certain events or feelings are happening. This begins in the dysfunctional family where we are given only the most rudimentary information about our circumstances, information which is often contrary to our own perceptions. The secrets, constant tension and repressive atmosphere in dysfunctional families give rise to denial.

A patient shared a good example of denial with me recently.

"I talked with my sister last night, Mary. I decided to tell her that my mother is an alcoholic, and share the book *Adult Children Of Alcoholics* by Janet Woititz with her. I figured she was already working on it herself. After all, she's a doctor. She denied the whole thing. 'That book has no relevance for us,' she said. 'Mom isn't an alcoholic. You know there's no such thing as a Jewish alcoholic.' She left me speechless, I can tell you. That line about Jewish alcoholics has been around our family forever. No wonder I've had to spend all these years working on my own denial . . . but I guess I shouldn't be surprised about that since no one in my family admits Mom's alcoholism even though she often passes out in the evening after she's had several drinks."

Some denial is normal for all of us, especially in certain situations. For example, denial is a normal stage in the working through of grief. If you've ever experienced the death of someone very close to you, you know how hard it is to believe that the person's never coming back. Patients with a terminal illness often deny the imminence of their own death until they have had a chance to process information and come to some acceptance.

But when families and individuals deny the realities of their daily lives, it distorts perceptions and leads people to distrust themselves. If Daddy is often drunk and you are always told he is "sick", you will feel that your judgment is faulty. Eventually, you will probably keep quiet and accept the family denial just to survive.

In some families all feelings and difficulties are denied and everyone looks well adjusted on the surface. If this is the case, there is usually one child who is forced to act out the painful feelings for everyone. He or she is the "identified patient" and has problems such as poor school performance, shoplifting, trouble with the law or depression. The rest of the family pretends to be normal and functions as if they have nothing to do with the child's problems.

Since denial is an unconscious process, you are usually unaware that it is influential in your life. Until you think, talk about and share your problems, you will continue to be blind to the role it plays.

Spouses often deny characteristics in one another when they are difficult or painful to face. Often, in fact, couples deny painful things about one another as a kind of exchange system: You can continue smoking a pack of unfiltered cigarettes a day as long as I can continue to use cocaine whenever I wish. I have patients just like this.

Guy is a computer graphic designer and Jean runs their small but busy office. Jean's habit is to inhale a little cocaine whenever she feels tired. Guy procures the cocaine for her and occasionally uses some himself. In an individual session Guy expressed concern to me about Jean's drug abuse, but he has never confronted her about it in spite of my suggestion that he do so. I was very puzzled about this until they began talking about her asthma and that of their youngest son. Then the basic bargain was exposed: I will let you smoke even though it is destructive to my physical condition (and that of our son) if you let me continue to abuse my substance of choice. Both Guy and Jean deny the harmful effects of cigarette smoking and cocaine abuse and the pattern continues.

This unspoken bargain is called collusion, which means that a destructive and unconscious pact is silently made between partners. Collusion is very common in co-dependent couples.

Compulsive Behaviors And Addictions

Dysfunctional families produce co-dependent individuals who are prone to addictions and compulsive behaviors. An addiction is the use of a substance or activity to medicate emotional pain. Our dysfunctional families teach us to look for happiness outside of ourselves and this, of course, leads to addiction and compulsive behaviors. Addiction consists of tolerance, which means that more and more of the substance is needed to produce the same effect, withdrawal symptoms when the substance is stopped and psychological dependence. In addition, there is compulsive ingestion of the substance. The most common substance addictions are alcohol, drugs (both prescription and non-prescription) and food.

Compulsive use is when you feel driven or compelled to ingest a substance or perform an activity. If you are compulsively using a substance or an activity to medicate your emotional pain, you feel out of control of the substance or activity. You can do almost anything compulsively: eat, gamble, have sex, spend money, horde things, practice religion and exercise.

If compulsive working is a problem for you, you will probably be reinforced, at least to some extent, by your community. Our society helps us to be driven about our work. It encourages monetary success and prestigious position. Compulsive working has become a pervasive, often unrecognized problem.

As we saw in Guy's and Jean's situation, compulsive behaviors are often a problem in marriages. Denial and collusion maintain these compulsive behaviors.

Grace and Richard are another good example of this. Both have been compulsive workers all of their lives and have formed several successful family businesses over the course of their working years. Both are now in their seventies and Grace is crippled by rheumatoid arthritis. Richard is still compulsively working, despite his age, and is gone every day from early morning until evening. Grace spends her days reading and drinking so that by the time Richard arrives home she is already intoxicated. Recently Grace was in the hospital for a minor procedure and began to exhibit signs of alcohol withdrawal (DTs).

Richard listened to Grace's doctor tell him about her withdrawal and the fact that her symptoms were indicative of alcoholism. He even communicated with his twin daughters about this, but by the next day he had concocted (in a purely unconscious way) a story about side effects from medication she was receiving. Grace was thus denied the opportunity to be confronted about her illness and perhaps to receive treatment.

There is a high degree of collusion operating here: Grace is tolerating Richard's compulsive working so that she can continue her addiction to alcohol. And Richard tolerates Grace's alcoholism so she won't confront him about his working and demand that he meet some of her needs for companionship and affection.

Poor Self-Esteem

Co-dependents have a poor opinion of themselves. Your self-image is formed by the feedback of others, starting in infancy. If you are a survivor of a dysfunctional family, you got little if any positive feedback about yourself. When children are held and cuddled and told how precious they are, they develop good self-esteem and know they are lovable. The opposite is true as well. If you are constantly corrected, criticized at every turn, called names, or physically abused, you will learn quickly that you are unlovable. If your parents don't love you, you wonder, who will?

This poor self-esteem will persist all of your life unless treated, and you will find yourself accepting abusive and negative behavior from others. Some authors call high tolerance for unacceptable behavior a characteristic of co-dependency. Poor self-esteem and abusive treatment are where this tolerance comes from. You will only accept abusive behavior from others if you have been treated abusively yourself or have watched a close family member be treated abusively. Abuse, if you are victimized by it long enough, becomes the norm.

Poor self-esteem also leads to depression, a pervasive and horrible feeling of helplessness and hopelessness. Although there is clear evidence that biochemistry and genetics play a part in depression, mental attitude and self-esteem also have a role.

In addition, and perhaps most significantly, poor self-esteem will rob you of your potential. You will never take risks because you expect to fail due to your poor self-image. Essentially, you will set a ceiling on your achievements the height of which will be determined by erroneous information about yourself.

Sometimes poor self-esteem masquerades as arrogance. In a co-dependent relationship this appears when one partner is always "wonderful" and the other is always wrong.

Michael and Betty were referred to me by her neurosurgeon after she had been hospitalized for a head injury she sustained during an automobile accident. Betty, in spite of her college education, had been assigned the role of "dumb bunny" in their marriage while Michael was thought of as wonderful and accomplished. This showed up in our first session:

"Tell me about yourself, Betty."

"There's nothing much to tell, Mary. Michael is the interesting one in our family."

"What Betty means is that she works for a small company in a little job. I am working for (names a large company) and soon I'll be promoted to management."

"Oh, are there plans for that in the near future? What's your position now, Michael?"

"I work in the warehouse, but not for long."

During this session, I asked Betty many more questions in which she deprecated herself and praised Michael. Their nonverbal behavior matched their verbal behavior: Michael strutted, Betty shuffled; Michael sat straight and spoke with authority; Betty slouched and stammered in a mild voice. Both denied there were self-esteem problems in their relationship. But in spite of their denial, it was clear that Betty was an underachiever who minimized her accomplishments in order to build Michael up. Unfortunately, they didn't come to their next appointment, perhaps because they were not ready to give up their collusion.

Boundary And Responsibility Problems

Boundaries form the limits of your personhood. They help you know where you begin and end, which thoughts are yours and which are someone else's, which feelings are your own and which belong to the person next to you. Co-dependent people have trouble with boundaries. They feel the confusion and sadness of others, and they take on responsibility for the well-being of other people in their lives. The trouble with this is that at best we have control only of ourselves, and then only to a limited extent. When we try to deal with another person's issues, we are doomed to failure. Responsibility and control issues are troublesome when boundaries are unclear and, it is my feeling, boundaries are the source of the trouble. Boundary disturbance is a key symptom of co-dependency.

Pauline Boss, quoted in *Facing Shame*, states that boundary ambiguity is "a state in which family members are uncertain in their perception about who is in or out of the family and who is performing what roles and tasks within the family system."

Fossum and Mason define boundary as "the ego barrier that guards an individual's inner space, the very means he or she employs for screening and interpreting the outside world and for modulating and regulating his or her interactions with that world. A person who grows up with clear boundaries can mature to a full and competent self. One cannot establish an identity without clearly defined boundaries."

In a dysfunctional family personal and interpersonal boundaries are vague and ambiguous and the continuous message to family members is that control is outside of the self. Survivors of the dysfunctional family then keep looking outside of themselves for fulfillment. Healthy families, in contrast, have clear boundaries and the locus of control is internal.

Locus of control is a very important thing, for if it is outside yourself, you look for security from things, substances and compulsive activities. You feel empty and look to others to fill you up. You have poor judgment because of repression and denial. If you are in charge of your own boundaries, or your locus of control is internal, you have clear judgment and all information is available to you because you haven't denied large chunks of it. You fill yourself and don't feel empty and you get security from your own thoughts, feelings, spirituality and relationships.

Table 3.1. Who Controls Your Boundaries?

Functional	Dysfunctional
You do	Others do
Internal locus of control	External locus of control
All information available	Denial deprives you of evaluating your situation based on all information
You feel full	You feel empty and needy
You rely on yourself, your relationships, spirituality, to meet your needs	You rely on others, substances, activities, to meet your needs

Symptoms of a boundary disturbance include:

- projecting or attributing your feelings to someone else
- blaming
- mind-reading
- fear of touching
- personalizing everything
- feeling confused when others are confused

- feeling "up" when others are "up"
- feeling "down" when others are "down".

There are several types of boundaries. The intellectual boundary contains and makes available your thoughts and knowledge; the emotional boundaries your feelings and the physical boundaries your body and its sensations. If you have experienced criticizing, blaming, prying or mind-reading, you have had your intellectual boundaries violated. If you were emotionally deprived or abandoned or if your parents shared inappropriately with you, your emotional boundaries were violated. Your physical boundaries were violated if there was incest, physical abuse or physical withdrawal.

Often boundary problems lead to responsibility and control problems. If you don't know where you end and I begin, and if you don't know who's in control of you, you will either be super-responsible and try to control everything or super-irresponsible and try to control nothing.

In close relationships, boundaries are particularly sticky. My patients, Jay and Connie, are a good example of what happens when boundaries are an issue within a relationship. For the 20 years of their marriage, they have been locked in a power struggle. Jay wants Connie to be sweet and nice at all times and looks to her to fulfill his needs. Connie wants Jay to be assertive but tender and wants him to meet all of her needs. Both try to tell the other what he or she is thinking, and their interactions are full of Connie's aggressive rage and Jay's passive rage. Well over one year of therapy was spent trying to separate them enough emotionally so that they could take responsibility for themselves and function independently. Each was so busy trying to get the other to meet all of their needs and take responsibility for all of the marital problems, that neither one was nurturing themselves.

Problems With Intimacy

Intimacy is a feeling state in which you feel safe and comfortable in a relationship, in which you know your partner will stay with you and attempt to understand and empathize with you. Intimacy presupposes knowledge, and in an intimate relationship you can allow yourself to be known for the very one you are, for all of your capacities and all of your incapacities.

You know when you are intimate with someone that you belong there. The relationship is your sheltering harbor. In it you can ride out the storms of your life, both internal and external and when necessary, you can sail away for a while, knowing your return is guaranteed.

According to Janet Woititz, you know you are in a healthy, intimate relationship when . . .

1. I can be me.
2. You can be you.
3. We can be us.
4. I can grow.
5. You can grow.
6. We can grow together.

She states further that,

> "Intimacy means that you have a love relationship with another person where you offer, and are offered, validation, understanding and a sense of being valued intellectually, emotionally and physically. The more you are willing to share and be shared with, the greater the degree of intimacy."
>
> *Struggle for Intimacy*

Sharing and exposure of self are wonderful experiences, but only in some situations. If you have exposed your emotional self over and over to people who treat you with hostility, rejection or indifference, you will learn to stop exposing yourself. Herein lies the problem for co-dependents from dysfunctional families. They have learned not to share in order to survive. Further, they were raised in a parental marriage which modeled dangerousness instead of safety, distance or fusion instead of healthy closeness.

If you have poor self-esteem, you will also be hesitant to share yourself for fear that the other person will find out just how very awful you are and reject you. So intimacy needs some level of self-love as a foundation. Without it, your confidence in love and acceptance from another person is shaky at best.

If you experienced invasion of your boundaries in your dysfunctional family of origin, you may confuse fusion with closeness and become terrified of closeness. Or you might strive for fusion because it is the only way you have been taught to fill the empty feelings inside. True intimacy is not empty but full, not scary but reassuring. Confusion in this area results in destructive relationships which further damage self-esteem.

If you have been in multiple failed and unsatisfying relationships and especially if they have all had the same problems in the area of closeness and intimacy, you need to look at what your pattern is expressing. Extreme and consistent distance in your family of origin will teach you to maintain distance from others and doom you to live a lonely and isolated life. Fusion in your early life will teach you to continually ask for inappropriate closeness in your present life.

Joe and Amanda have a relationship which looks wonderful on the surface, but if you spend any time with them, you sense a tremendous emptiness. In spite of their obvious material success, both are lonely and depressed. Amanda is on a constant round of social activities and Joe is a compulsive worker who finds life a continual trial. The death of Amanda's younger brother brought her into therapy:

"I'm so upset I don't know what to do or where to turn. Jack was only 37 . . . I could talk to him and I miss him terribly."

"What will you do about talking about your feelings now?"

"I don't know. That's why I'm here, Mary. I realize that Joe doesn't care to talk about feelings and all of my

so-called friends change the subject when I try to talk
about Jack. I'm so lonely."

Amanda's grief and tears did a lot to expose her to the
realities of her life, and Joe joined her in therapy some
months later. Both are still working on building intimacy
in their marriage.

Depression & Anxiety

Co-dependents are prone to feelings of depression and
anxiety and these often occur together. Depression
consists most commonly of a loss of interest or pleasure
in usually pleasurable activities, appetite and sleep
disturbance, decreased energy, difficulty concentrating,
negative thoughts, and irritability. Anxiety shows itself
in motor tension or restlessness, physical signs (such as
sweating, dry mouth, pounding heart), worry, appre-
hension and hyper-alertness.

Ira and Jean each have many of these characteristics,
and their relationship magnifies them. Jean is chronically
depressed and negative about the state of the world.
Having a conversation with her is like visiting a shelter
for the homeless: you come out depressed. Ira is just as
negative and he is a compulsive worrier with long-
standing insomnia. Her negativity plays into his worry.

"I didn't sleep at all last night. I'm so tired . . ."

"Well, what do you expect, Ira. The news last night
says it all . . . The situation in the Persian Gulf will kill
us all and that little girl on her third liver transplant. I
wonder why they torture her that way. Why not let her
die . . . we all will, anyway."

"The other thing is money. You have been spending
way too much on shoes again, Jean. I wish you would
stop it!" (Jean has more closets in her house than most of
us have rooms and all of them are full of shoes.)

This conversation goes on all the time Jean and Ira are
together in endless negative variation. Is it any wonder
they are both depressed and complain of having no
friends?

Most co-dependents are anxious and depressed. This can be attributed to post-traumatic stress syndrome from growing up in a dysfunctional family. Post-traumatic stress syndrome is composed, according to the American Psychiatric Association, of the following:

1. The history of a stressor which would evoke symptoms of distress in anyone
2. Re-experiencing the trauma with
   - recurrent recollections of traumatic events
   - dreams about stressful incidents
   - sudden, intrusive feelings that the events are happening again in the present because of an associated environmental stimulus
3. Numbing of responsiveness
4. Several of the following:
   - hyper-alertness
   - sleep disturbance
   - survivor guilt
   - trouble concentrating or memory impairment
   - avoidance of activities which remind one of the original trauma
   - symptoms increase with repeated exposure to memories of the traumatic events.

Dysfunctional families are like a war zone. People get hurt both emotionally and physically and there is no end in sight. Your goal becomes survival. There is no one to talk with about what is happening. And the difficult and painful feelings go on and on and on . . . In a situation like this, people develop the symptoms of co-dependency and post-traumatic stress syndrome. Then they bring those symptoms into their relationships to continue the cycle.

Stress-Related Illness

Many illnesses are known to be stress related but I'm sure we haven't even begun to get the full picture yet. In the future, more and more diseases will be known to have occurred or worsened because of stress. Hypertension, headaches, gastro-intestinal diseases, heart disease, multiple sclerosis and even cancer have so far been attributed, at least partially, to stress.

Often co-dependent people have symptoms of these illnesses and co-dependent relationships are focused on the illness. Dave and Cheryl, for example, are dealing constantly with Dave's ulcerative colitis. Ulcerative colitis can be a life-threatening illness but Dave is irresponsible about his treatment and medication and refuses to follow the diet which has been prescribed for him. So Cheryl hovers over him, giving him his medicine, and grilling him about his diet. Both are so focused on his illness that they address no other issues. Their sexual relationship is non-existent and both are depressed and feel needy because no communication goes on between them except for that which focuses on Dave's colitis.

Co-dependency, as you can see, is a serious disorder which affects many of our lives. It contaminates relationships and sabotages the self. Co-dependent characteristics lead us into certain types of intimate relationships. Although the prototypes we look at here are by no means the only forms co-dependent relationships take, they represent a general range. Table 3.2 summarizes and contrasts co-dependency in the individual and within a relationship.

Table 3.2. Co-dependency Characteristics:
Alone And In Relationships

Co-dependent Individual	Co-dependent Relationship
Denial — denies important parts of own history or present reality	Relationship denial or collusion — couple denies information about each other ("You really don't eat, smoke, drink, work too much") or relationship exchanges ("You can smoke if I can use cocaine".) Many couples pretend they are close in spite of feeling empty and distant.
Compulsive behaviors and addictions	Individuals bring these to their relationships, where they use problems to justify their own addictive behavior ("I wouldn't drink so much if you were more supportive".)
Poor self-esteem	Both partners usually have this, sometimes it shows up as a "good" and "bad" partner.
Boundary and responsibility issues, "Where do I end and you begin?"	Partners feel each other's feelings, read each other's minds, try to control each other's behavior.
Problems with intimacy	Either fused or distant; many myths and stereotypes in the relationship ("All men only want one thing".) ("Women should be barefoot and pregnant".) Maintain the perfect facade, even if you feel empty.
Depression and anxiety	Relationship is depressed, isolated, negative; both worry about what the other is feeling.
Stress-related illnesses	These occur in the relationship, when both people are needy and sometimes illness is the only way to get nurtured. Stress of relationship causes illness.

4
PATTERNS
IN THE
CO-DEPENDENT
MARRIAGE

There are many forms of co-dependent marriages, but the examples used here are the most typical. Of course, specifics vary from relationship to relationship, but we often (more often than we like to admit) fall into recurrent patterns of interaction. These patterns usually have their roots in our dysfunctional families. Each pattern includes a table comparing co-dependent characteristics and their place in the marriage.

All of the cases used are composites based on real people but disguised to protect privacy. The marital patterns are described in no special order. Look for yourself in the sections which sound familiar. You may find that you identify with more than one section.

Abuser/Victim: Cheryl and Robert

She perched like a terrified exotic bird, rigid and vigilant, on the edge of my soft overstuffed chair. She had blonde hair, long and wavy and was well dressed but very tense. She seemed to know it was time to tell the secrets, but she was afraid. Tears coursed down her face.

"You won't tell anyone, will you, Mary?"

"No. But you do need to talk. It's important so you can get better." This spoken softly with the acknowledgment of her fear.

"He beats me. Robert beats me and it's getting worse." Cheryl was sobbing now, sound wrenching involuntarily from her throat.

"Tell me about the beatings. How often and about what?"

The story was told over several sessions. Cheryl's husband of three years beat her regularly with his hands, fists and feet. And it was getting worse — more frequent.

The beatings followed a pattern: Robert would arrive home from work shortly after Cheryl. Some nights their interaction was bland, even pleasant. Those evenings they would eat the dinner she had prepared, Cheryl would wash dishes, and they would sit together and watch television. Then they would go to bed, perhaps even make love.

But this was less and less the pattern. More often than not, Robert would come home and act irritable, be demanding. Cheryl would respond to his demands with increasing tension, trying to please him but knowing she couldn't.

After one or several evenings of vicious verbal abuse, the battering would start and, over a period of 10 days or so, would escalate until Cheryl was hurt. Then the apologies began and for a few days Cheryl and Robert laughed and loved together until the whole terrifying cycle repeated itself.

One day Cheryl arrived for her session more visibly upset than usual. In the waiting room she faced away from me when I came out of my office to get her, then turned to expose an eggplant colored eye and jaw and a deeply lacerated, swollen lip.

"Good grief, Cheryl . . . are you all right? What happened?" Her face looked terrible. Hearing about the beatings was one thing, seeing such graphic evidence another.

"He's been madder and madder all week . . . upset that I'm seeing you. He's worried about work. It's been building for a few days. He tried to choke me this time." We were standing inside my office by now, and Cheryl gingerly opened the ruffled collar of her blouse. Blue marks curled around her slender neck. I almost cried.

"Please, Cheryl, I know we haven't known each other long, but you have to get out of there, at least for a few days. Did you lose consciousness? Was he still mad after the beating was over?" My questions, while jumbled, were an attempt to judge how seriously she had been injured, and where Cheryl and Robert were in their pattern . . . if there would be any more beatings.

"I stayed conscious most of the time, but for a while things went black. And he's still angry today. He called at lunchtime and yelled at me."

"You simply have to get out of there now."

"But I have no money and nowhere to go."

"There's Safehouse. Do you know about Safehouse? It's a shelter where battered women can go when they need to escape from their houses for a while. I don't know where it is because that's a secret, but we can call someone to pick you up."

Cheryl agreed that her life was in danger if she returned home that night. The call was made, and I loaned her ten dollars for cigarettes. She left to meet the Safehouse staff member, and promised to call if I could help her further. But my next call was from Robert.

"I know Cheryl has been seeing you and she went to the Safehouse on your advice. She won't need to go there again because I'm going to get some help. I don't know what's wrong with me but you can just tell her to come back home. It's only happened a few times . . . I just lost control."

In spite of his satin voice, he sounded dangerous to me. "I understand that this has been happening for several years and that it's been getting worse."

"No, no. Cheryl exaggerates. Only a few times. Really. I've hardly hit her at all."

"How dare you say 'hardly any violence' when Cheryl's face was battered purple and your fingermarks showed around her throat? If you really wanted to get help, you'd take responsibility for what you've done."

Those comments exposed my anger and probably disqualified me from doing couples therapy with Cheryl and Robert. I must confess, however, that I really wasn't worried about that at the time. My thoughts were much more with Cheryl, bruised and alone, hiding in the Safehouse in fear of her life. Robert hung up on me that day, and it would be five years before I would hear from Cheryl again.

1986

My answering service gave me a message to call Cheryl, which I did.

"I don't know if you remember me, Mary. We saw each other a few times in 1981. I'd like to see you again."

She arrived for her appointment wearing a business suit, tastefully made up with her hair its natural brown color. The first thing she did was pay back the ten dollars she had borrowed from me years ago.

In 1983 she had left Robert, finally and irrevocably. Cheryl had been picking up the pieces since then. During five years of severe marital violence, and in spite of a Master's degree in business, she had only been able to manage a receptionist's job in a quiet office.

"It was as if he took away my soul. The physical beatings weren't the worst, because the emotional abuse left me with very little of myself. There was a broken arm, broken ribs and collarbone, and several head injuries. But he kept choking me, which is what finally convinced me that Robert would murder me if I stayed with him."

Cheryl and I worked together for several years. Over the course of time, it became clear that both she and Robert had come from very dysfunctional families.

Cheryl explained that Robert's father deserted his family when he was four years old. His mother gave up at that time and never recovered, becoming more and more depressed as Robert grew up. Robert was raised without attention and nurturing. His mother fed and clothed him, struggling all the while, but she was unable to relate to him emotionally.

I formed a mental picture of a small boy playing by himself in the corner of a crowded and dirty apartment. Although I had never met Robert, it was clear from what Cheryl said that he grew up with the idea that women are victims, and that he was not worthy of love and attention. His own sense of deprivation must have generated profound rage, which he suppressed until he found someone upon whom he could vent it.

The more Cheryl and I talked, the more obvious it became that Robert's problem, as well as her own, was related to co-dependency. Robert's symptoms, in addition to his rage and low self-esteem, included severe anxiety over his own work performance and attempts to control Cheryl with physical and emotional abuse.

Cheryl came from a different type of dysfunctional family. She was the youngest child and only girl in a prosperous farm family. Although her family attended church and were active in community affairs, her father physically abused her two older brothers and verbally abused her and her mother. Because Cheryl's mother allowed her sons to be physically abused and herself and her daughter to be emotionally battered, Cheryl also came to see women as the passive victims of tyrannical men. All of the abuse in Cheryl's family was a secret. Her father made it clear that if anyone outside the family learned how he behaved, the children would be treated even more brutally.

"I remember standing behind a tree in one of the fields one day watching my brothers help my father set fence posts. He was very angry at them for something they weren't doing properly and he shouted obscenities at them. No one knew I was standing there, and if I moved I would have been discovered. So I stood and watched while he got madder and madder. Finally he hit Randy so hard that he was left lying on the ground gasping for breath. Josh tried to stop him, but he couldn't. I thought Randy was seriously hurt, but he just got up and started working again as soon as he could."

"How old were you, then?"

"I was nine or ten. The boys were older . . . thirteen and fifteen."

When Cheryl watched her brothers abused, she, like other children in the same situation, expected her turn to come. Children's terror in this situation profoundly affects their later life. They become ever vigilant, waiting for their own beatings. Cheryl also learned to see men as violent and unstoppable. That knowledge, combined with her mother's example of secrecy and denial and her poor self-esteem (which had its beginning in her father's belittling), set her up to marry an abusive man and to play the role of his victim.

Robert and Cheryl had evidence of a problem during their engagement. Robert slapped Cheryl after an argument. He apologized profusely and promised that it would never happen again. Both denied the significance of the incident and both kept it secret.

Robert and Cheryl, because of each of their histories, thought that one person, usually the man, should be in charge of the relationship. Neither could talk about feelings. Robert, enraged because of his early abandonments (father left physically, mother emotionally . . . he lost both parents at the same time) stuffed his feelings down until intimacy with a non-perfect (read human) woman brought them out with all their destructive potential.

Cheryl, convinced (by her mother's collusion in and acceptance of her children's abuse) that women are victims, thought herself helpless. Her family of origin was so conscious of appearances that she learned never to ask for help or confide in others. She left Robert when her denial finally broke down and she realized her life was in danger. As is typical in violent marriages, the violence would have become worse with the passage of years, especially if no one had got treatment.

Cheryl was able to leave Robert before she was killed. She has recovered from her catastrophic experiences to the extent that she is able to work effectively and now enjoys her life. One problem still remains. Cheryl is unable to commit herself to another intimate relationship.

Abusive relationships usually have their own cycle in which tension, anger and rage gradually build up. This culminates in one or several battering incidents, and finally a making up or honeymoon phase takes place. Power inequities are the norm in battering relationships and one partner, usually the abusive man, makes all of the decisions for the couple. There is often life-threatening denial of the seriousness of the battering behavior. Such behavior never gets better without intensive treatment. Violence sometimes escalates to murder.

Physical abuse, while it is the most dramatic and visible, is not the only kind of abuse which takes place in relationships. Sexual abuse often accompanies the physical abuse in violent marriages and emotional abuse is universal in these relationships. As Cheryl told me, the emotional abuse can often be the most destructive behavior because it undermines self-confidence so much that the victim finds herself unable to believe she can succeed in living without the batterer. Some marriages have no physical or sexual abuse but emotional abuse is a daily occurrence. These relationships must also be thought of as abusive and violent. The same issues which operate in the abuser/victim relationship operate in an emotionally abusive relationship.

The abuser/victim pattern is not confined to heterosexual relationships. It occurs in homosexual relationships as well. Of course, the real rate of abuse within relationships is difficult to ascertain because both the victim and the abuser have tremendous feelings of shame about the violence.

Learned helplessness is another common phenomenon in abusive relationships. According to Lenore Walker, a well known researcher and writer in the field, this is the reason many victims never leave their abuser. Learned helplessness is developed after repeated unsuccessful attempts to control the events in our lives. With the consistent inability to influence outcomes, we become more and more depressed and passive. Ms. Walker describes one experiment which vividly illustrates how learned helplessness works:

> "Newborn rats were held in the experimenter's hand until all voluntary escape movements ceased. They were then released. This procedure was then repeated several more times. The rats were then placed in a vat of water. Within 30 minutes, the rats subjected to the learned helplessness behavior drowned. Many did not even attempt to swim and sank to the bottom of the vat immediately. Untreated rats could swim up to 60 hours before drowning. The sense of powerlessness was generalized from squirming in order to escape handholding to swimming in order to escape death. Since the rats were all physically capable of learning to swim to stay alive, it was the psychological effect of learned helplessness which was theorized to explain the rats' behavior."

It seems to me that for those of us who grew up in dysfunctional families, learned helplessness begins very early when we learn we are unable to influence Mother's drinking or drug abuse and/or Father's sexual abuse or workaholism. This consistent early experience generalizes into a rest-of-my-life pattern and we feel unable to influence outcomes across the board.

This inability is then carried into marriage, where it is easy to get locked into behaviors which reinforce our helplessness. Cheryl learned she was unable to change her father's verbal abuse of her and his physical abuse of her brothers. She carried this lesson into her marriage to Robert where each violent incident reinforced it. Soon she became emotionally paralyzed.

Abuser/victim is only one example of the co-dependent marriage. It, like all the other types, is built on low self-esteem, isolation, inability to communicate feelings and denial. The marital positions seen in the abuser/victim marriage are enmeshed and controlling. Table 4.1. illustrates co-dependent characteristics in the abuser/victim relationship.

Table 4.1. Co-dependency Characteristics And Abuser/Victim Relationships

Co-dependency	Abuser/Victim Relationships
Compulsions • destructive, "driven", • serve to distract from pain	Rage attacks: abuser is driven, destructive, distracted from pain. Victim is distracted from her pain, self-destructive.
• alcohol abuse	Alcohol is often implicated in violence.
Power/Control issues • co-dependents think they can control others or can be controlled by abuser	Abuser: tries to control victim. Victim: is controlled by abuser; changes her life to please him/avoid violence.
Anxiety/depression	Both have symptoms.
Poor self-esteem	Both have symptoms.
Boundary disturbances	Abuser: violates victim's physical boundaries with abuse. Victim: allows own boundaries to be violated
Responsibility issues	Abuser: blames others for actions. Victim: accepts blame for abuser's actions.
Health problems	Abuser and Victim suffer from severe stress and psycho-physiological symptoms.
Denial	Of life-threatening injuries.

Silent Type/Loudmouth: Hilary and Bruce

It was getting dark outside, the early winter darkness which falls like a shroud over frozen snowy streets. And Hilary's voice was droning steadily. I wondered if she ever paused for breath. A short cap of dark hair framed an attractive blue-eyed, creamy skinned face. But in spite of her obvious intelligence and pretty appearance, I wanted to sleep, to shut out the annoying voice.

I was taught that the best therapists use their own feelings as a gauge to tell them what is happening with clients, and with this woman I had to force myself to stay awake, in spite of the fact that doing therapy is usually fascinating to me. My sleepiness and sense of boredom meant that Hilary was very depressed, or perhaps that she was extremely passive-aggressive.

Passive-aggressive behavior is that which expresses anger without being obvious. Chronic lateness for appointments, always forgetting insurance forms or checkbook, calling late in the evening with inconsequential problems and canceling appointments at the last minute are some examples of passive-aggressive behavior in therapy, and it's hard to confront these behaviors because there are always seemingly unassailable excuses. Any anger is vigorously denied. If Hilary was being passive-aggressive, it was a form I had not often seen: constant talking. She had called for an appointment several days prior to our interview and she had told me that her main problem was depression which she attributed to her long-standing 24-year marriage to Bruce.

During our phone conversation she said she had been struggling with severe depression for over 10 years and was on antidepressants which were prescribed by her family physician. She had in the past seen various therapists and once was hospitalized for her depression. She was 45 years old and her youngest child, a 17-year-old girl, was to leave for college the following fall. Her two sons had already established themselves independently; one was in the Navy, one was a college graduate married and living in a different state. Hilary's husband Bruce was a salesman for a large computer manufacturer and traveled a great deal.

"The problem is in the marriage, Mary," she told me in my office during our first session. "Bruce just doesn't give anything at all. When he is home, he just sits there and watches television. I have help in the house, but I work full time and I shouldn't have to do it all: the cooking, shopping, laundry and all the work with our daughter. We have no sex life, no social life and he won't talk to me. I just can't do it all alone anymore, Mary."

As her voice continued its litany of complaints, I was reflecting. Usually I would be the first to side with any woman who said she had to do everything at home and work full time, but I could see that something else was going on here.

I interrupted Hilary's monologue by asking her about her family of origin. The middle child in a wealthy family of seven, she grew up in New England and attended boarding school and college there. She was raised by a series of nannys until being sent to boarding school at the age of 14. Her parents maintained very separate lives. Her father was absorbed in the family business, her mother in social and community events. In short, no one paid attention to Hilary. She met Bruce when they were both in college and married shortly after graduation because Hilary was pregnant. The early years of the marriage went well and were busy with three small children and Bruce's growing career. The family moved every two years or so as Bruce was given different sales territories and responsibilities. When the children were all in school, Hilary returned to college and earned her graduate degree in Library Science. By then the marriage was already beginning to sour.

"We never had much of a sex life, at least not so I could enjoy it. I think Bruce has always had a problem with premature ejaculation. No matter how hard I've tried, he has never got help with it, and when I was in my 30s, we had sex about once every two weeks. I insisted on more sex, but the more I asked for, the less Bruce would have and now we don't have sex at all.

"When the children were small, he would do a few activities with them, especially the boys, and we made some friends that way and through my efforts in the neighborhood. Now I see my friends, but he won't join me . . ."

I had to interrupt Hilary three times to close her session, but we finally scheduled another appointment and she left my office. I was exhausted and relieved that she was my last patient of the day. Our next two sessions were much the same: Hilary talked constantly, absorbed none of my feedback and had to be repeatedly reminded that time was up. I left each session fatigued and feeling drained. I had learned very little, except that Hilary was needy, unhappy and self-centered. Enter Bruce.

Twenty minutes late for our first couple's session, he shook hands with me, smiled, accepted my offer of water, apologized for being late and sat in his chair with the longest, loudest sigh of resignation I have heard before or since. If I was looking for passive-aggression, I had found it.

"Do you always sigh like that?" I asked.

"Did I sigh? I wasn't aware of it."

"Yes, Mary, he always sighs like that, and then he denies it. I think it's terrible. He just won't talk to me about anything, and there's no affection. All Bruce does is earn money and watch television . . .". Hilary was off on another tirade. She never raised her voice, but she monopolized, criticized and put Bruce down for as long as I would let her. After one couple session, I made an appointment to see Bruce alone.

"I don't think there's any hope, Mary. I want a divorce. I can't stand to live there. All I hear is criticism and demands. I'm a very successful man at everything except my marriage to Hilary, and there I'm a miserable failure."

"Tell me about some of your successes, Bruce."

"I have been promoted to district manager of my company and my earnings are in the six figures. In spite of what Hilary thinks, I have good relationships with my sons. I talk to them on the phone every week or more, and manage to visit about every third month. She's ruined our daughter by always putting me down, and I don't have a relationship with her, a fact I regret very much."

"What about friends?"

"I have lots of friends at work and several in other parts of the country. I can't make relationships as a couple because people can't stand to be with Hilary for long. She talks too much, and all of it is negative."

"Have you ever talked to her about this?"

"Until I'm blue in the face, but she doesn't listen, doesn't hear. And I know I don't hear her either. I've been trying to tune her out for so long."

"What about the withdrawal of affection and sex?"

"I would always ejaculate too soon, and she would always let me know about it, loud and clear. It got worse and worse and finally I stopped trying. I don't have that problem with anyone else."

"Anyone else?," I said, with unconcealed surprise. "Have you been involved with other women?"

"'For a long time I was faithful to Hilary, but finally I had a relationship with a woman and discovered I could satisfy another person, and that I wouldn't have to listen to all that endless criticism . . . I think it has saved my life really."

"Does Hilary know, Bruce?"

"No, although I don't try to hide it too much. She doesn't seem to want to know."

This case ended unhappily: Bruce and Hilary did get divorced and Hilary did not stay in therapy long enough to benefit from it. Bruce didn't come back after the divorce was filed.

I have, over the years, seen several cases like this. They're a kind of cliche in which the woman (usually) does all the talking and all the expression of emotion for both members of the relationship, but also takes all the heat. While I was treating Bruce and Hilary, I knew nothing about co-dependency. Since then I have learned about it and now co-dependency seems a particularly appropriate concept to apply to relationships like this. Both members of the relationship blamed the other for their unhappiness, both denied the importance of Bruce's affairs, both were enmeshed in compulsive behaviors.

Maggie Scarf in *Intimate Partners*, calls this type of relationship "a classical system". She points out that the silent husband in this system is afraid of emotions and the hysterical wife is afraid of her own emptiness. She further states that ". . . even when he does consent to hear her out, he does so with little or no empathy. What she says rarely penetrates the self-protective armor he wears . . . The more she emotes, the less he listens; and the less he listens, the more . . . emotive she becomes."

Other authors (Stahmann and Hiebert) state that partners in this type of relationship want to lean on each other and be taken care of, but view their dependency needs with distaste and both pretend these needs are not there. They also cite the prevalence of poor self-concept and sexual difficulties in these relationships.

Peter Martin in *A Marital Therapy Manual* describes this type of relationship as "The Love 'Sick' Wife and the 'Cold Sick' Husband". "The wife," he states, "comes for therapy first because she has been experiencing severe anxiety, depression or incapacitating physical symptoms . . . she claims her symptoms are entirely due to the coldness or cruelty of her husband. She insists he does not care about what she wants or what she feels." He continues to describe the wife in this marital pattern as a person who blames her situation on her husband's inadequacies. "To her, the only solution is a change in her husband."

The husbands in these relationships, while competent and successful in their professional lives, often fare badly in their relationships. "Some were unable to show feelings of closeness, intimacy, anger or love . . . They suffered from the problem of intimacy in close relationships. They had fixed, rigid character structures . . ." (Martin).

How, I always wondered when I came across such couples, did two such different people come together? The answer seems to lie, once again, in the traditional analytic concept of projective identification.

According to Maggie Scarf in *Intimate Partners*,

"... projective identification has to do with one person — say me — seeing my own denied and suppressed wishes, needs, emotions, etc., in my intimate partner and not experiencing those wishes and feelings as anything coming from within my own self. If, for instance, I were a 'never angry' person, I might see anger as coming only from my husband — and actually get him to collude in this by forcing him to lose his temper and express my anger for me . . .

"Intimate partners often perform this function for each other: experience and express what are actually the spouse's unacknowledged and repudiated emotions. When one person is always angry and the other is never angry, it can be assumed that the angry spouse is carrying the anger for the pair of them. And similarly, when one partner is very competent and the other nonfunctional (depressed, for example), there is usually an unconscious deal in effect, a collusion about who will take ownership of which particular feelings."

Co-dependency can certainly flourish in a marital relationship in which the partners are denying their feelings and making each other responsible for the expression of them. In all silent type/loudmouth relationships there is a lot of anger operating but it is on an unconscious level and the partners may not be aware of it.

It often looks like one person makes all the decisions for the pair but this itself is a joint decision in that the silent partner refuses to make decisions. The loudmouth is blamed if there are mistakes. Sometimes, too, there is a quiet but effective acting out on the part of the silent partner using money, guilt or compulsive behaviors against the loudmouth. This serves to passively express his or her anger and sabotage the partner.

The resolution of this type of marital conflict involves each partner taking responsibility for himself and all of his feelings.

> "This means learning to experience ambivalence — the good and the bad within the other and the good and the bad within the self. It involves, in plain words, seeing both one's goodness and one's badness, one's craziness and one's saneness, one's adequacy and inadequacy, one's depression and one's happy feelings, etc., as aspects of internal experience . . ."
>
> *Scarf*

Table 4.2. Co-dependency Characteristics and Silent Type/Loudmouth Relationships

Co-dependency	Silent Type/Loudmouth Relationships
Compulsions • destructive • distract from pain	Compulsive talking and working keep each partner from focusing on issues.
Anxiety/Depression	Usually the "Loudmouth" expresses these for both.
Poor self-esteem	Both partners have this.
Responsibility Problems	Blame each other for marital dissatisfaction; project feelings on one another
Problems with Intimacy	Separate friends, no affection, poor communication.
Denial	Of destructive elements in the marriage (affairs, the effects of constant talking) Of own feelings

Triangles or Three's A Crowd: Carolyn and Bob

The anger in my office was palpable. Carolyn, a tall, slender, blonde woman in her late 30s was red-faced and gripping the arms of her chair.

"Unless you set some limits on that child, I'll leave you. She has no right to disrupt my marriage and my home and you are so weak you can't make any decisions, so I have to make them. I want her to shape up."

"You have no business saying what my daughter does. She's 18 and she can make her own decisions." While he was more controlled, Bob was obviously enraged too. His fists were clenched in his lap and his bright blue eyes glittered with emotion.

This fight was one in a long series of disagreements which began to surface when Bob's daughter (from his previous marriage) had come to live with Bob and Carolyn for her first year of college. My original patient was Carolyn, who had been working in individual therapy on her depression and family of origin issues. But Katie's presence in their household had precipitated so much conflict that Carolyn and Bob were seeing me together.

"You think she can make her own decisions, do you? Then why did she use such bad judgment that she drank herself into a stupor and then proceeded to drive her car off the road? Why did she let that man follow her into a deserted parking lot . . . and all the other things she does? She acts like a silent, sneaky ghost when I'm around, but I'll bet she hangs on you when I'm not. And you talk more to Katie these days than you do to me. Our marriage is being destroyed and she's begging you for limits which you won't set. She'll end up killing herself in her car if you don't do something."

There was a real problem with Katie in that she was acting out and covertly asking for structure and Bob was not giving her any. But the power struggle between her and Carolyn wasn't entirely Katie's and Bob's fault. Carolyn's family of origin had set up this scenario long before Carolyn was capable of logical thought.

Carolyn's parents both came from dysfunctional families and, when their first child (a son) was born, Carolyn's mother bonded to him immediately, to the exclusion of her rather narcissistic husband (this was the first triangle in Carolyn's family:)

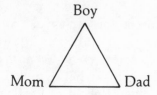

He, in turn, took Carolyn over when she was born to create a polarized family (this was the second triangle:)

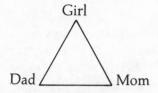

Carolyn was the youngest child, a girl, and she was used as the scapegoat in the family. Her parents fought over and with her constantly. Her mother rejected Carolyn, and her father, feeling rejected himself, gathered her closer until he became angry with his wife, at which point he lashed out at Carolyn. Her brother tried to support her but was only able to do so covertly. He did not want to jeopardize his hero status. Carolyn had been in triangles all of her life. Now Katie was helping her act out another one.

There were several other triangles which operated in Bob's and Carolyn's marriage before Katie came on the scene. These were all engineered unconsciously by Carolyn to keep her intimacy with Bob at a tolerable level. She had one very close female friend in whom she confided far more than she confided in Bob and a senior colleague with whom she related as if he were her father. Both of these relationships prevented Bob from getting too close to her. She was terrified of being hurt.

Bob was baffled by Carolyn's other relationships and felt somewhat hurt because they took her away from him, but he denied the significance of her friendships from which he was largely excluded. He turned to alcohol, which he drank on a nightly basis to medicate his anxiety and loneliness. Bob and Carolyn, in spite of these shadowy triangles, felt they enjoyed much of their marriage until Katie moved in.

Every parent knows that if there's a chink in the armor, a teen-ager will widen it until it is a split. Katie sensed the problem and, herself a survivor of a dysfunctional family, maximized it. In addition, she legitimately wanted fair and firm limits which, of course, she was unable to ask for directly. The fewer limits Bob would set for her, the more she acted out her anger. If Carolyn stepped in and tried to direct her, Bob passively undermined her efforts.

Bob wanted his daughter's love and felt guilty about having to abandon her when he, in spite of his best efforts to make their marriage work, divorced Katie's mother. Katie and Bob had maintained a close relationship in spite of their distance (Katie and her mother had moved to another state) and prior to living with Bob and Carolyn, Katie had seemed to be developing a relationship with Carolyn as well.

But now after eight months in their home, Katie had succeeded in adding fuel to an already smoldering fire.

"Don't you see, Bob. We have to do something before she hurts herself or tears our marriage apart . . ." now Carolyn was sobbing.

"This is so hard," Bob said, looking worried. "I want Katie to be happy, but I want you to be happy, too." He turned to me with a helpless gesture. "What can we do, Mary?"

"I suggest we keep talking about both of your feelings and that we look at creating a contract with Katie which compromises on everyone's needs."

Over the course of several sessions, we discussed what should be included in the contract. Katie was invited to attend therapy with Bob and Carolyn but she refused. The contract which was finally presented to her included some limits, some privileges and a deadline on how long she could continue to live in Bob and Carolyn's household. But the issue of triangulation remained.

Triangles generally occur when one or both partners is frightened of intimacy or have difficulty with trust. In a relationship in which there are two participants, intimacy can grow and increase, but when three people are in a relationship, intimacy gets diluted and each individual feels less vulnerable.

According to Guerin *et al*, "Understanding triangles and triangulation in marital conflict is essential to identifying the dyfsunctional process in marriage and mapping out appropriate intervention."

There are several ways triangles can operate within marriage. In one type of triangle, the spouse who is most uncomfortable and upset recruits a third person to relieve tension and give support. (Carolyn's friend and colleague are examples of this.) Another type of triangle "involves a third person (often a child) who is sensitized either to intensive conflict in the relationship or to anxiety in one spouse. The third person moves in to calm the upset or is caught up in the process and acts out in some way." (Guerin *et al*)

If you come as Carolyn did from a family in which you were used as part of a destructive marital triangle, your tendency would be to repeat the dynamics of your family of origin. Triangulation would then become a pattern in your own marriage.

Triangles also allow a marriage to continue without change. Carolyn and Bob would have been forced to confront their own marital issues before Katie moved in with them had it not been for Carolyn's supportive friend and colleague. "The third person," according to Maggie Scarf, "provides a middle alternative — a way of dealing with the difficulties other than the starker options of facing the problems and dealing with them directly or of ending the marriage completely." They also, of course, allow distance and dilute stress within the marriage. The third person often gives the couple an issue upon which to displace their conflict.

The extramarital affair is one of the most common and destructive forms of triangulation.

> "An affair can have any of several effects on a couple. It can calm the uncomfortable spouse without disturbing the other spouse, thus stabilizing the marriage and covering over its dysfunction. But this effect is often temporary and usually ends when the other spouse finds out about the affair. Then the affair itself becomes the central issue between the spouses, again covering over the conflictual process in the marriage that triggered the affair in the first place."
>
> Guerin *et al*

Another particularly destructive form of triangulation occurs when a child is a part of the marital triangle. Children are casualties of the marriages in which they are used as a scapegoat, as Carolyn was in her family of origin. Here the scapegoat child is the repository of all the rage and disappointment of her parents. Often these children behave in the ways they are treated and develop poor self-esteem and emotional problems. And as we saw with Katie, Carolyn and Bob, "It is often easier for marital partners to discuss (or fight wildly about) the intolerable behavior of a child than it is to discuss feelings of rage, grief, disappointment and discontent about the relationship they share." (Maggie Scarf)

The concept of triangulation in marriage teaches us still more about co-dependent relationships. The central issues are again co-dependent ones. All three of the marital positions: enmeshed, detached and controlling appear in triangular marriages.

Table 4.3. Co-dependency In Triangulated Relationships

Co-dependency	Triangles
Compulsions • destructive, driven • distract from pain	Add third parties to close relationships to distract self from vulnerability and fear.
Power/Control Issues	Try to maintain control by diluting involvement.
Anxiety/depression	Both have symptoms.
Poor self-esteem	Both have symptoms.
Boundary disturbances	Often try to maintain firmly closed boundaries (walls) with third party acting as a buffer.
Responsibility issues	Both blame third party or each other.
Denial	Of own problems, of destructive nature of behavior.

Doctor/Patient: Carmen and Joe

A pale narrow face, dark eyes and pixieish brown hair were all that showed from beneath the white hospital sheets. This was my second visit to Carmen, whose neurologist had asked me to consult. She had a potentially deadly diagnosis: rule out multiple sclerosis. (The "rule out" diagnosis means that a particular illness is suspected on the basis of the person's symptoms. The patient is usually given a diagnostic work up for that specific condition. Because multiple sclerosis, a gradually progressive and debilitating disease which attacks the nervous systems is an illness for which it is difficult to establish a firm diagnosis, the "rule out" diagnosis is often applied over long periods of time.)

It was Carmen's third admission to the hospital with numbness in her legs and feet and headaches. Both the nursing staff and the physician felt there was something not quite right in Carmen's life. Something she wasn't talking about and maybe was not aware of. One of the nurses had mentioned Carmen's husband Joe as a potential problem, but she really couldn't put her finger on what it was that had made her uncomfortable.

"How are you today, Carmen?"

"I'm okay. How are you?"

"Doing well, thank you. Where did we leave off . . . I think you said you had been in the hospital two other times with numbness. When was that?"

"In the past year."

"In between episodes you're fine, right? What do you do?"

"I work in an office. I've had my job for four years, and I really like it. I do all the books and word processing for a small manufacturer."

"Any hobbies?"

"I used to run, but I don't do that anymore. I do some needlepoint."

"Tell me how long you've been married. How is your husband taking all this?"

"We've been married about a year and a half, and Joe couldn't be sweeter about my being sick. He brings me flowers and new nightgowns and even a teddy bear . . . I feel so lucky that he's so nice."

Our conversation continued on a fairly superficial level, but a few things struck me. Carmen did not seem at all anxious about her symptoms or about the possibility of having MS. If I had been in her shoes, I would have been very anxious, very depressed or both. The timing of her symptoms bothered me, too. She had been married for over a year, and her symptoms had started shortly after her marriage. Multiple sclerosis is known to be made worse by stress. So I wondered was her marriage stressful on some level?

Our interviews continued throughout her five-day hospitalization, but in spite of my probing, I could learn very little about what was going on with her emotionally. Everything was usually just fine. I encouraged her to come for out-patient appointments, but she didn't follow through. A few months later, she was hospitalized again. Her symptoms were identical, and her physician still could not pin down a diagnosis. He asked me to consult again and fortunately my schedule forced me to visit in the evening. Joe was there.

"It's nice to finally meet you, Mary. Carmen's told me a lot about you."

"Nice to meet you, too, Joe. How are you, Carmen?"

"I think she's going to be all right, Mary. Aren't you, hon? It's hard for us while she's sick, but she'll get better. Do you need anything . . . some water, or a piece of candy?"

Something was drastically wrong here. I'd been in the room for several minutes, and Carmen hadn't put a word in edgewise. Joe, an attractive dark-haired man, was hovering constantly, answering questions for her and talking nonstop in a very anxious manner. I hardly heard Carmen's voice until I sent Joe out of the room for something. "Does he always act like that?" I asked her with a smile. "He seems worried to death."

"Yes, isn't it wonderful!" she smiled back. "I love being taken care of."

It takes something incredible to render me speechless, but that just about did it. Taken care of is one thing, but smothered is a whole new level. There was definitely something strange going on here. I spent an hour in Carmen's room that evening while Joe paced and brought pillows and water and helped Carmen to the bathroom as if she were 80. I grew more and more confused.

The next day I asked some very specific questions of Carmen and what I learned provided the beginning of my understanding of this marriage. Carmen did all the work in the marriage. She cooked and cleaned and washed and ironed and she earned the bulk of the income because Joe's sales job paid on a commission basis. Joe made all the decisions on how money was spent even though he earned only a small part of the household's total. If he did earn a commission, he generally bought himself something he wanted, such as a new camera or some clothes for himself. Carmen was forced to work overtime to earn extra money. Even if Joe was home, which he often was, he did none of the household chores and no cooking. Carmen would come home from work, cook dinner and clean up. On weekends she did laundry and cleaned house. Sometimes Joe helped with vacuuming, but the rest was her job. Joe's family lived in town, and the couple's social life usually centered around them.

They were also active in their church, and Joe, especially, volunteered for several extra activities and committees. Carmen didn't have the time or the energy to devote to others. Everyone liked Carmen and Joe. No one had yet seen what really went on in their relationship. Fortunately, in this case, both partners were willing to enter therapy on the premise that if stress wasn't causing Carmen's illness, it was at least making it worse.

Joe was the only male in his family of origin. His father died shortly after he was born and he was raised by his mother and two older sisters. Joe simply never thought to do the household work. At home that was his sisters' and mother's domain. He was catered to, picked up after and fed his favorite foods. No one ever pointed out to him that he was the only member of the family not working in the house. Joe's mother and sisters coddled and petted him and he took no responsibility for anything. After high school he attended a local college, but never finished his degree. He lived at home earning a little money from his sales job. Whatever money he earned, he spent on his car or on his dates and social activities. No money of his went back into the household.

Carmen was the only child of an alcoholic mother and a distant father. She ran the household from a very early age when her mother became less and less able to function. Carmen was used to going to school all day and coming home and cooking a meal and doing dishes. Her childhood had been spent trying to keep her family together and cover up her mother's drinking. She left home after high school but continued to visit and try to add some order to her mother's life. Tragically, shortly after Carmen moved out, her mother was killed in the house, the victim of a fire which apparently started from an unattended cigarette. (I wonder what message she got from her mother's death. Do people die when you separate from them and stop working on their behalf?)

This marriage continued the dynamics each lived in their families: Carmen was working herself to death without recognition and Joe was accepting this as his due and contributing nothing. Carmen, in spite of this, denied her marital problems. Instead of confronting them and demanding the attention and help she needed, she converted her issues into physical symptoms.

There was fortunately a catch. Joe loved Carmen and it frightened him when she was ill. He showered her with TLC, flowers and candy and that was the only nurturing Carmen got. This could have produced continued and worsening symptoms, rendering Carmen a cripple with a life-destroying psychological illness. Joe and Carmen, I am happy to say, worked hard together to share responsibility and learn to nurture each other and themselves. Their marriage has blossomed as a result.

Some doctor/patient relationships don't end as happily. Sometimes the "nice guy" doctor really gives nothing emotionally but looks wonderful on the surface. Underneath he or she is cruel, demeaning, destructive but "takes care of" his or her crippled partner. Both partners in this relationship are needy. The doctor gets plenty of accolades from friends and family and lots of support from the community while worsening, in effect, the patient's illness. The only way the patient gets anything from the relationship is by continuing to be ill.

> "Since (the) symptoms are a product of stress, deriving from denied, ill-defined or unacknowledged marital conflict, (the patient) will now . . . be caught in the circular process of illness-confirming behavior . . . symptoms will gradually become a displaced focus for marital conflicts and dissatisfactions. Instead of grappling with issues of power and control in the marriage . . . symptoms (can be used) to exercise some power indirectly."
>
> *Hafner*

Joe's and Carmen's relationship illustrates one type of doctor/patient relationship, the type which develops in response to unmet needs in the marriage. Another type of doctor/patient relationship occurs because of the illness or disability of one spouse. This is the marriage in which one partner is needy and dependent and the other a professional caretaker. (In fact, this happens frequently in the marriages of physicians, nurses and therapists who are literally professional caretakers.)

You may get involved with someone who is ill, addicted or disabled because you have learned in your family of origin to take care of others instead of being cared for yourself. The premise can be succinctly stated, "If I just give enough, maybe I'll get something." In this type of relationship, caretaking allows the caretaker to maintain control in the relationship. With caretaking comes the unspoken position that it is acceptable for the caretaker to hide his or her inner self on the theory that one is acceptable as long as one is unknown. No one could love me if they really knew who I am so I must control how much they know about me, as well as their behavior.

Robin Norwood states this dilemma clearly in *Women Who Love Too Much:*

"When efforts to help are practiced by people who come from unhappy backgrounds or who are in stressful relationships in the present, the need to control must always be suspected. When we do for another what he can do for himself, when we plan another's future or daily activities, when we prompt, advise, remind, warn or cajole another person who is not a young child, when we cannot bear for him to face the consequences of his actions, so we either try to change his actions or avert their consequences, this is controlling. Our hope is that if we can control him, then we can control our own feelings where our life touches his . . .

"A woman who habitually practices denial and control will be drawn into situations demanding these traits. Denial, by keeping her out of touch with the reality of her circumstances and her feelings about those circumstances, will lead her into relationships fraught with difficulty. She will then employ all her skills at helping/ controlling in order to make the situation more tolerable, all the while denying how bad it really is. Denial feeds the need to control and the inevitable failure to control feeds the need to deny."

(Ms. Norwood uses the feminine pronoun, as her book is directed to a female readership, but I believe this applies equally to both sexes.)

Like other co-dependent relationships, doctor/patient relationships enmesh people in pathology in their desperation for a sense of belonging and love. Denial, control problems and poor self-esteem are at the heart of the matter again. Marital positions commonly seen in doctor/patient relationships are enmeshed and controlling.

Table 4.4. Co-dependent Characteristics and Doctor/Patient Relationships

Co-dependency	Doctor/Patient Relationships
Compulsions • destructive, driven • serve to distract from pain	To care for others. To control others.
Denial	Of marital problems.
Power/Control Issues	Control with illness or caretaking.
Anxiety/Depression	Both have these.
Poor self-esteem	Both have this.
Boundary disturbances	Who is in charge?
Responsibility Issues	Who takes responsibility for health?
Health problems	Symptoms as a result of unmet needs in the relationship or the stress of constant caretaking.

Please Note: It is not necessarily a doctor/patient relationship when one partner is ill but takes responsibility for his/her own recovery and rehabilitation. In the normal course of events in a couple's relationship, each will help the other with illness, but recovery is the primary responsibility of the person who is sick.

The Merger Relationship: Judy and Stan

I have always liked working in hospitals and when I maintained a full-time practice, I was often asked to consult for medical and surgical patients. The gratifying part of those consultations was being able to work with people who might otherwise never seek therapy. Stan and Judy were people who, despite their severely co-dependent marriage, had no insight whatsoever into their marital problems.

The consultation request came from an orthopedic surgeon and the nursing staff. Stan had been involved in an automobile accident in which he had crushed his leg. This 42-year-old man, a very successful independent insurance agent, had been hospitalized for almost a month and had undergone three surgeries to stabilize his critical fractures. He was understandably worn out and depressed when I met him.

A tall, spare man with shaggy salt-and-pepper hair, Stan greeted me with a noticeable lack of enthusiasm. His long legs, one of which was encased in a heavy cast, seemed to overflow the length of his bed. His face was grey and drawn. This long and painful illness and all the medications he was taking had sapped him completely by this time. Still he would discuss only his feelings about his wife and her situation.

"I'm really worried about her. And I miss spending time with her. She doesn't drive so she has to depend on other people to bring her to the hospital, and she's running out of food at home. And she's so lonely. We do everything together and it's terrible to be separated. I want you to see if you can help her."

"What about you, Stan?" I asked with some concern. Surely he was suffering most of the stress in this situation. He had horrible pain and he had been confined to the hospital for a long time. (This long a hospital stay is very unusual now, but Stan's was a very complicated orthopedic problem which took place some years ago.)

"I'm not having too much trouble except for missing Judy. She's the one who's suffering."

He had no sooner finished his sentence when Judy walked in. A large woman, she looked barely pulled together. Her yellow hair showed long dark roots and was every-which-way, her clothes were attractive but mismatched and while she smiled at her husband, she seemed lost . . . as if she had wandered into the wrong room.

"Hello, love. How's your leg today? I got a ride with Lynn, so I can stay till late. I'll have to take a cab home anyway." Judy paused to be introduced to me, then went back to her conversation with Stan. "I hope you're in less pain. Sometimes I swear my leg hurts too. Did you sleep? I'm so worried about you and I can't stand to be separated like this. We've only been apart for one night in the 21 years of our marriage until now, and I miss him so much". Her eyes had filled with tears, and Stan was visibly disturbed, too.

"Honey, please don't cry. I hate to see you so upset. You know I'd be home if I could. In fact, Doctor Lawrence says it will probably only be another week to 10 days." Their visit continued with occasional questions from me. Observing Stan and Judy brought to mind that destructive description of a marital partner, "the better half". They looked very much like half people who needed each other to be complete. Instead of a marriage they had created a merger.

In the plant and animal world, symbiosis is a word which describes mutual beneficial dependence. In marriages, the same mutual dependency when carried to extremes is destructive and parasitic. The partners live off each other. Stan's and Judy's marriage was a good illustration of this. They had married in their early 20s and both were children of dysfunctional families. Judy lived with her mother's chronic mental illness and repeated institutionalization and Stan had been raised by his elderly and rigid grandparents after the death of his father when he was eight. His mother had died giving birth to him. They saw each other as life rafts. They attached to one another like barnacles to the hull of a ship, firmly and permanently.

Judy stopped driving early in the marriage and was therefore dependent on Stan to drive her everywhere. Although she at first had a job independent of Stan, as his insurance business built up, Judy worked more and more in his office and finally gave up her job altogether. For many years they had worked in the same office in their home, gone shopping together, done household tasks together, gone on vacation together and spent almost every waking and sleeping moment together. Stan sometimes had business appointments without Judy, but she usually accompanied him. Neither had hobbies other than symphony attendance and movie-going. Those they did together. They saw very few other people because they were "too busy" and they had no children. They rated their marriage as wonderful. They stated they had very few conflicts and neither would acknowledge the faults of the other or admit to feeling smothered.

I had reason to question their happiness. Although I articulated very little of my concern, my probing yielded denial and more denial. Stan had been severely hyper-tensive for many years and Judy had incapacitating headaches. They were so focused on each other that neither attended to their own life issues and problems. Their rather restricted life style sounded like a prison to me and although I worked with them in a supportive way for several months, their marriage remained too close, a fusion which allowed little individual develop-ment.

Merger relationships begin when both partners are deprived of basic caretaking and nurturing as children. Often these relationships take the form of relationship addictions.

"In love addiction, the ties of dependency run from one partner's inner child to the other's inner child. Something within addictive lovers makes them believe they need to be attached to someone in order to survive, and that the other has the magical ability to make them whole. This is why love often goes wrong. Addictive lovers don't believe they can be whole alone."

Brenda Schaeffer

The issues of aloneness and dependency are a core struggle in the marital relationship. In mature love relationships, each partner is allowed to lean on the other when necessary, but both are encouraged to be independent and to fulfill many of their own needs. In contrast to the mature marriage are the marriages of people like Judy and Stan, people labeled in psychiatric parlance as passive dependents.

Scott Peck in *Road Less Traveled* discusses them eloquently:

"People with this disorder . . . are so busy seeking to be loved that they have no energy left to love . . . They tolerate loneliness very poorly. Because of their lack of wholeness they have no real sense of identity, and they define themselves solely by their relationships . . . it is one of the behavioral hallmarks of passive dependent people in marriage that their role differentiation is rigid, and they seek to increase rather than diminish mutual dependency so as to make marriage more, rather than less of a trap . . . By so doing, in the name of what they call love but what is really dependency, they diminish their own and each other's freedom and stature. Occasionally . . . passive dependent people when married will actually forsake skills that they had gained before marriage."

Peck goes on to give the example of a wife who gives up driving when she is married, or even well into the marriage. "The effect of this . . .", he states, "is to render her almost totally dependent on her husband and chain her husband to her by her helplessness . . . Because this behavior usually gratifies the dependency needs of both spouses, it is almost never seen as sick or as a problem to be solved . . ."

Merger behavior comes from the deeply entrenched sense that there is not enough, that I am not enough. And this invariably comes from the lack of consistent nurturing and love in early childhood. The healthy bonding in marriage turns, in these circumstances, to rigid and destructive, albeit denied, bondage.

Jurg Willi in *Couples in Collusion* calls this "dyadic fusion: the partners form a symbiotic union or a mutual self . . . this may lead to excessive intimacy and loss of ego boundaries, dissolution of the self . . . (Often) an image of inviolable seclusion is presented to the outside world." The couple is isolated and still more firmly entrenched in their pathological dependency.

As you can see, of course, boundary problems are at the bottom of fusion. You give yourself up to another only when you don't feel separate, strong and lovable within yourself. A person like that resembles the proverbial Dutch boy with his finger in the dike. He inadequately but desperately holds himself together until he is flooded by the tides of intimacy. Then the dike breaks down and the self is carried away. In merger relationships, the primary marital position is entrenched.

Table 4.5. Co-dependency Characteristics and Merger Relationships

Co-dependency	Merger Relationships
Compulsions • destructive, driven • serve to distract from pain	To be together, to fuse.
Power/Control issues	Neither has control of life; the relationship engulfs them both.
Anxiety/depression	Often both have symptoms.
Poor self-esteem	Both have poor self-esteem.
Boundary disturbances	Merged boundaries, no clear identities as individuals.
Responsibility issues	Each takes responsibility for each other and the relationship, but not for self.
Health problems	Common.
Denial	Of problems.

The Arm's Length Marriage: Abby and Greg

Abby's long black hair gleamed blue in the sunlight. Her round body slumped a little in my chair. "I don't know what's wrong but when he's home, we fight all the time and when he's gone, I miss him terribly. I'm relieved when he leaves, but by the second day I hate him for letting me cope with things all alone."

Greg was a busy and successful salesman for a national clothing company. His work kept him on the road for five days almost every week. Abby had two small children to care for and she worked part-time in a local department store. She called me for treatment of her depression.

"Greg is my third husband and I'm beginning to think I wasn't cut out for marriage. The first two were a lot worse, especially the second. He was violent and drank. The first time I was pregnant and too young to know better . . ."

Greg and Abby had been married for four years. Greg had always traveled quite a bit, but a promotion two years after their marriage had increased his time on the road. He had accepted the promotion without consulting Abby. There was nothing unusual about that, according to Abby, as Greg made all of his decisions without her input and did exactly as he wished with his time and energy.

Greg's unilateral decision-making had angered Abby more and more, and her resentment showed in the increasing number of arguments between them. Although they spoke with one another on the phone every evening, this was not enough contact to maintain the sense of intimacy so necessary in a marriage.

"By the time Greg comes home, I'm so miserable and so exhausted that I fight with him even more. I don't know how to stop it."

"Tell me about your family. Where did you grow up?"

"I was raised in Chicago. My father was a trucker, and he was killed in an accident when I was very small. For years my mother has been involved with a man named Ray . . . she's never married him, thank goodness, because that would change her insurance benefits from my dad's accident. He's mean and has beaten her several times. He used to scare me a lot, and I always wonder if my mother will be all right. I'm an only child."

Abby's small family was certainly dysfunctional given the early death of her father and her mother's later violent relationship. Abby had become pregnant right after high school and married the father of her baby, only to find herself trapped at home with a small child, no career and a husband who spent more time with "the boys" than with her and their baby. Abby and her first husband were divorced after two years of a marriage which sounded suspiciously like her present marriage: distant.

After two years of working, Abby met her second husband and she replaced an empty and distant relationship with another replete with turmoil, alcohol and violence. Her marriage to her second husband ended after less than a year. She had met Greg about two years later, and married him after a year of courtship. Their son was now three years old.

Greg came in to see me a week later. A tall, handsome man with bright red hair and turquoise eyes, his stance and muscular definition made it clear he was a body-builder. It was difficult to engage him in conversation as he was suspicious and a little angry that Abby had already spoken with me.

He had been raised on an isolated farm in Nebraska. His parents had been strict and rigid and showed very little affection. His marriage to Abby was his first.

"I really don't know what she wants from me. It seems like whatever I do isn't enough. I don't think I can spend more time with her. After all, my job keeps me on the road four or five nights a week and there are things to do when I come home."

"Like what?"

"Well, the cars always need work and the lawn. I go to the gym to catch up on my workouts and we see friends.

Then the whole thing starts over and I'm back on the road. We talk on the phone every night, but lately I've been tempted not to call because all we do is fight."

Abby, Greg, and I worked together for several months. They would alternately fight and discuss his distance and her loneliness. We all discussed the human tendency to relive our parents' marriages. Both were very motivated to continue their marriage on a more intimate level. Greg took a job which required less travel, modified his compulsive exercise routines and they made more time alone together and with their children.

Greg is still working on his capacity for intimacy and Abby is still working on her anger and trust issues. Their marriage, I am happy to report, has shown every sign of improvement.

The arm's length marriage is common when one partner (or both) travels a lot or when both partners are troubled by intimacy and closeness. Why do people maintain such detached relationships? The primary reason to maintain an arm's length marriage is the fear of intimacy.

The first issue here is the fear, based on poor self-esteem, that once someone gets to know me, they will find me unlovable. This fear, in reality a firm internal belief, leads to the fear of abandonment. And the fear of abandonment is virtually universal in those of us who survived a dysfunctional family.

Abandonment takes place on a physical level, that is when parents aren't there physically to meet the needs of the child, and on an emotional level. Emotional abandonment is as traumatic as physical abandonment and it includes passive neglect as well as abuse of any kind. (A patient once told me one of the worst stories about abandonment I ever heard. Her uncle, as a small child, came home from school one day to discover that his family had left the house and the town without him. They had literally moved away while he was in school. Some days later, the school authorities found him, crouched and soiled, in a corner of the house. He had no food, no heat and no electricity. This kind of thing probably happens more often than we know.)

Abandonment fears keep us in relationships which are destructive because loss frightens us above all. And they keep us from allowing our relationships to be intimate for fear that, once we are known, we will get left. Without the feeling that we are lovable, we are doomed to the lifetime of emptiness and distance symbolized by the arm's length marriage. In this type of relationship we see the hallmarks of co-dependency: poor self-esteem, compulsive behaviors and issues around intimacy and closeness. Detachment is the usual marital position in these relationships.

Table 4.6. Co-dependent Characteristics and The Arm's Length Marriage

Co-dependency	Arm's Length Relationship
Compulsions • destructive, driven • serve to distract from pain	Compulsive exercise, relation-ship addiction.
Power/Control issues	Often unilateral decision-making.
Anxiety/Depression	Both
Poor self-esteem	Both
Boundary disturbances	Too distant, keep from being vulnerable.
Responsibility issues	Who should work on relation-ship? How much to risk?
Health problems	Often.
Denial	Of issues, of feelings.

Addict/Addict: Laura and Duane

In spite of the spring freshness in the air and the sunlight streaming through my office windows, the young man looked strained and desperate. His carefully arranged sandy blonde hair contrasted with his clothing, which was rumpled and stained. Duane was an emergency room physician who had just left the hospital after working all night.

"I'm so angry at Laura I can hardly stand to go home anymore. I work harder and harder and she spends more and more money. We are in debt now, and I'm not sure I can get us out of it this time . . . she keeps opening new charge accounts. I make a lot of money, but she spends all of it and more. Every time I turn around, there's something new in the house . . . something major like a large screen TV or a new dining room table. I've tried to take the charge accounts away from her and hide the checkbook, but she always finds a way around it . . . What am I going to do?"

Duane and Laura had been married for four years, and this problem had been getting worse. They had met while Duane was a resident in a large hospital in Dallas. Laura had been a speech pathologist in the same hospital. For the first two years of their marriage, both had worked. When they moved to Denver where Duane had secured an emergency room position, Laura quit work, "just until the house was fixed up", and the excess spending started. Two years later, Laura still had not returned to work. Duane's continued efforts to control her had been unsuccessful.

At my insistence and in spite of the fact that he found it easier to focus on Laura, Duane told me a little about himself. The only child of a small town family practitioner, Duane had always known he would someday be a doctor. His mother was a quiet woman who kept a spotless home, fresh baked goods, and who waited slavishly on her husband and son. She had no interests of her own and on reflection sounded rather depressed.

Duane's father was usually gone on rounds in the small community hospital where he practiced or in his office. Everyone loved him but Duane never got to know him. Now as he talked some of his childhood loneliness was expressed for the first time.

"I never questioned it at the time, but Dad was never home. I played by myself when I was very small, then made friends in school and spent a lot of time with them at their homes. Their Dads were around a lot more. Some of them even spent time playing baseball with us. My mother worked in our house all the time. She was a wonderful cook and the place was always spotless, but she was rarely still. When she did sit down, she was quilting or doing needlework of some kind. I used to want her to color with me or read to me, but she never would . . ."

Isolation was evident throughout Duane's life. He went from a secluded little boy to a man whose energy was always focused on work or on the hard-driving competitive study required by his top-notch college and medical school. His relationships had, until his marriage, been mostly social and superficial. He admitted he had his share of difficulty with intimacy.

I saw Laura the next day. Her dark hair was stylishly cut, her makeup flawless and her casual clothing whispered money. She didn't want to be in my office.

"I'm only here because Duane says he'll get a divorce if I don't come. There's nothing wrong with me except I'm lonesome . . . Duane's gone all hours of the day and night, and I'm alone. There's nothing to do except watch TV . . . all my family is still in Texas, and I have only made a few friends here. I think he expects me to wait on him like his mother did and I won't do it!"

"Duane's told me he's upset about the way you spend money, but before we get to that I'd like to ask what you think is going on in the marriage."

"Well, that's the point, not much. Duane works 12-hour shifts in the emergency room, and he's gone a lot at meetings and things . . . not much happens between us anymore. We fight about money and he wonders what I do all day, but we don't talk much anymore. Once in a while we go out with another doctor and his wife, but usually he's too tired to do anything."

"What about sex?"

"What sex? We don't have much sex anymore."

"Don't you feel abandoned?"

"Yes, I guess I do."

Laura came from a large and wealthy Texas family. But her father, in spite of his material success, was an alcoholic. Her mother played the role of a "social butterfly" and the children pretended nothing was wrong, except for Laura's older brother, who committed suicide when he was 18. He had been the family's identified patient until his death. Now that role belonged to a younger sister who was drinking, using drugs and had recently been caught shoplifting.

Both people from dysfunctional families had found each other. Together they made another kind of co-dependent marriage. Duane was addicted to work and Laura was addicted to spending money. Later it also became clear that she was bulimic and addicted to eating binges and purges. Although our society sanctions addiction to work, especially in a physician or other health care professional, compulsive work still serves to fill up an internal emptiness and to distract from emotional issues.

If addiction is "a pathological relationship to an activity or substance" (World Health Organization), then work can certainly be addictive. As is usual in addict/addict marriages, Duane and Laura blamed each other for their addictive behavior. Duane in effect said that if Laura wouldn't spend so much money, he wouldn't have to work so hard. Laura then accused Duane of neglecting her and spent money to soothe her feelings of abandonment.

Compulsive spending is a surprisingly common habit in our culture. Shopping malls and charge accounts are so usual they occasion no comment, and many people are caught in the effort to fill their internal emptiness with material goods. As you can see, this is simply another way to avoid feelings and to call on external resources to solve problems.

Bulimia as well as the other eating disorders (compulsive overeating, anorexia nervosa and thin fats) are still another example of using a substance to dull feelings and thoughts and to turn us away from our internal selves. Because obesity is socially unacceptable, Laura's bulimia allowed her the illusion of control over her compulsive overeating. But purging becomes in the situation as addictive as eating. Bulimia is an expression of the control/release cycles inherent in all addictions.

Laura was a typical bulimic; she was thinness focused, had a distorted body image (she saw herself as fat) and she was perfectionistic with poor self-esteem. Her compulsive buying and her eating disorder gave her instant gratification and a way to escape her bad feelings.

Addict/addict relationships take place between any two kinds of addicts. Although we usually think of two alcoholics at the bar or two heroin addicts spinning dreams together, addiction is a very common problem in our middle and upper classes.

You can be addicted to anything. In fact, according to Anne Wilson Schaef,

"An addiction is any process over which we are powerless. It takes control of us, causing us to do and think things that are inconsistent with our personal values and leading us to become more compulsive and obsessive. A sure sign of an addiction is the sudden need to deceive ourselves and others to lie, deny and cover up. An addiction is anything we feel tempted to lie about . . . An addiction keeps us unaware of what is going on inside us. We do not have to deal with our anger, pain, depression, confusion or even our joy and love because we do not feel them, or feel them only vaguely . . . As we lose contact with ourselves, we also lose contact with others and the world around us. An addiction dulls and distorts the world around us . . . (and) our sensory input. We do not receive information clearly; we do not process it accurately and we do not feed it back or respond to it with precision. Since we are not in touch with ourselves, we present a distorted self to the world . . . and (we) eventually lose the ability to be intimate with others, even those we are closest to and love the most . . . An addiction (also) absolves us from taking responsibility for our lives . . ."

When Society Becomes an Addict

In addition, poor self-esteem forms the foundation for every kind of addiction.

"Most addictionologists agree that low self-regard is a crucial factor in all forms of addiction. The chronic absence of good feelings about oneself provokes a dependence on mood-changing activity. Manifest or masked, feelings of low self-esteem are basic to most dysfunctional lifestyles . . . (because) one way of coping with disquieting factors is to immerse oneself in an activity that is incompatible with serious self-evaluation."

Milkman and Sunderwirth

In addition to poor self-esteem and obsessiveness, addiction has a cycle, a predictable sequence of its own. Although the following information is paraphrased from Patrick Carnes' *Out of the Shadows*, a profound work on sexual addiction, this cycle is relevant for every type of addiction.

The first phase of the addiction cycle is the preoccupation with the substance or activity to which you are addicted. You enter a mood, a kind of trance, wherein your mind is taken up with thoughts of your activity or substance. This is followed by a ritual composed of activities or thoughts which intensify your preoccupation and which lead up to your addictive behavior. The behavior itself comes next, behavior which you feel unable to stop or control in any way. The end of the cycle is the shame and despair, the feelings of hopelessness, and the promise to yourself that the behavior will never happen again. This cycle occurs in all addiction, but only after you have acknowledged the destructive nature of your behavior. Denial of the problem will prevent the awareness of the cycle and the final sense of shame.

We can see co-dependency operating in the denial of feelings, responsibility issues and poor self-esteem of both partners in the addict/addict marriage. These relationships are usually enmeshed and controlling.

Table 4.7. Co-dependency Characteristics and Addict/Addict Relationships

Co-dependency	Addict/Addict
Compulsions • destructive, driven • serve to distract from pain	Work, money, binges
Power/Control issues	Who controls working, spending
Anxiety/depression	Both
Poor self-esteem	Both
Boundary disturbances	Each takes other's behavior as a reflection of self
Responsibility issues	Each tries to control and be responsible for other
Health problems	Frequent, especially at end stages of addiction
Denial	Of feelings, problems, addiction itself

Addict/Enabler: Melissa and Jim

The tall balding man sitting opposite seemed to me to be a plodder; that particular type of individual without whom most of us would be lost. He would stand, I imagined, behind the scenes, doing whatever had to be done and in a timely, efficient manner. I felt no connection, even after seeing him several times, to his emotions.

Jim had come to me because of his concern for his wife, Melissa. She had been resisting therapy and so far would not come to see me with him.

He described a difficult situation: He and Melissa had a three-year-old son, and two months before they had had twin girls. The enormous amount of work and the continuous demands of the children had apparently taxed her to the limits of her tolerance. Melissa stayed at home and did very little most of the day.

"I don't know what she does, Mary. On weekends, when I'm home, she mostly stays in bed . . . she says she's exhausted. I can't understand it, although I know the babies are tough . . . I try to help."

"What do you do to help out?" I asked, thinking maybe the problem was simply that what he thought was help wasn't helpful enough.

"Before I go to work, I feed the girls and make sure Jason has breakfast. While Melissa rests, I dress all the kids . . . I try to get home at lunch and feed the kids again, and change them, too. I put them down for their naps when I leave. Then, when I get home, I feed them again, bathe them and put them to sleep. I read Jason a story and put him to bed, too. Then I try to fix us some dinner or order pizza and straighten up the house, maybe do some laundry. I think I help as much as possible."

"Good grief, so do I!" I was appalled. "What does Melissa do while you're at work?"

"I don't know. The kids are always wet and dirty when I get home. Sometimes Melissa makes an effort to clean the house, but usually she's still in her nightgown at lunch and in sweats at dinner. She doesn't do her hair anymore unless I nag her."

"I think it's time you told her she has to come in here. She sounds so depressed that I'm beginning to think she'll need to be hospitalized." I was thinking about the possibility that Melissa was suffering from post-partum depression, a severe mood disorder which results from a combination of hormonal and emotional factors soon after delivery. Jim and I scheduled an appointment and he agreed to bring Melissa even if she continued to resist.

When I met Melissa, I was relieved that I had insisted on seeing her. She was more emaciated than petite and her pallor and the dark circles under her eyes spoke of her depression. After learning that Melissa was the child of two alcoholic parents and that she did, in fact, feel at the end of her resources, we discussed how child care arrangements could be made so that she could be hospitalized. Our goals were to work with her depressive emotions but also to have consultation from a psychiatrist in order that she start on anti-depressant medications. It seemed straight-forward enough.

It was straight-forward until Melissa's second day in the hospital when she had her first *grand mal* seizure (convulsion). Afterwards, when her mind was clear again, Melissa admitted she had been taking Valium. Although she had denied drug use both during our interview and upon admission to the hospital, her seizure frightened her enough to break down her denial. That was fortunate, because sudden withdrawal from Valium can produce uncontrollable seizures which sometimes cause death.

"My obstetrician prescribed the Valium when I couldn't sleep after the twins were born, and I just kept refilling the prescription. I had no idea they were addictive, but they made me feel so much better. After a while, I started drinking wine with them, and that helped even more. I wouldn't get mad at the babies or at Jason, and I didn't think I could get into trouble with it, Mary, really." Jim had no idea she was using Valium and, while he saw her taking an occasional glass of wine, he saw no difficulty with that. How much denial and collusion was going on in this marriage? And how much enabling?

Enabling means that one partner passively allows the other to avoid the consequences of his or her behavior. In this case, Jim allowed Melissa to be nonfunctional for several months by taking over all of her responsibilities and not confronting her about her behavior. In this way her depression and her dual addictions could be denied, but she lost the opportunity for early treatment as well. Still since Jim took over child care, Melissa was under little pressure to deal with her drug abuse and her depression. This is the essence of enabling — the enabler allows the addict to get away with his or her addiction. We all know that change requires effort and pain, so if there are no consequences of dysfunctional or irresponsible behavior, why change?

There are lots of varieties of enabling. If you are the enabler in your relationship, you might clean up your addict's messes (such as broken dishes from a drunken spree or a child's disappointment that a commitment was broken), cover up for your addict when the effects of his or her substance interfere with functioning, hide the substance, and take over the responsibilities of the addict, as Jim repeatedly did for Melissa. Enabling makes the addict's addiction your problem, too.

Patrick Carnes, in *Out of the Shadows* describes it well:

> "Enabling, in contrast to controlling, stems from denial and rationalization. Covering up for the addict, protecting him or her from consequences and keeping silent about personal concerns are the behavioral ingredients of enabling. It involves a fundamental dishonesty which entails insane denial of what one knows to be true."

Enabling means the system allows the addict to maintain his addiction by colluding with him and pretending it's not a problem. Enabling sometimes looks like helping, but it isn't . . . not for the addict and not for the enabler.

Enabling often involves very dysfunctional behaviors on the part of the enabler. These commonly include:

- disregarding one's own intentions
- overlooking hurtful behavior
- covering up behavior which one despises
- appearing cheerful in spite of hurt
- avoiding conflicts to keep up appearances
- allowing oneself to be repeatedly disrespected
- allowing one's own standards to be compromised
- faulting oneself for family problems
- believing one has no option.

Patrick Carnes

Enabling helps the addict stay addicted and ruins the enabler's life as well.

In Melissa's case the physician who repeatedly refilled her Valium prescription played an enabling role in her addiction. His failure to warn her of the drug's addictive potential and his continuation of her prescription gave her the message that her drug use was acceptable. This is often the case with drugs like Valium, other minor tranquilizers and sleeping pills. Always ask your physician whether the drug you are taking is addictive. Then look it up, in order to double-check your information in a consumer medication guide or ask your pharmacist.

The problem isn't only the doctors and the husbands and wives of addicts or alcoholics. The problem is our society, in which we are taught to ignore difficult and uncomfortable emotions and behavior. This pattern of denial helps people stay hooked on drugs, alcohol, sex, food and other behaviors and substances. Addict/enabler relationships have all of the hallmarks of co-dependency. Denial and responsibility issues head the list and enmeshment is the usual marital position in these relationships.

Table 4.8. Co-dependency Characteristics and
Addict/Enabler Relationships

Co-dependency	Addict/Enabler
Compulsions • destructive, driven • serve to distract from pain	Substance and controlling use and consequences of addiction
Power/Control issues	Who's in charge? Enabler tries to control addict
Anxiety/depression	Both
Poor self-esteem	Both
Boundary disturbances	Whose feelings are whose?
Responsibility Issues	Enabler takes all responsibility, addict takes none
Health Problems	Addict, from substance; enabler, from stress
Denial	Both deny seriousness of problems

5
RECOVERY
AND
TREATMENT

The goals of recovery are, essentially, to make your life rewarding, rich, satisfying and fun. And to help you be the best person you can be: open, warm, flexible and self-loving.

Recovery

There are many definitions of recovery: Recovery is not perfection, but growth; it is not a destination, but a journey. And, I must add, a journey which is not often smooth, in which you will have to face things which are unpleasant and difficult. In other words, recovery is a process which will require growth and change and openness and the ability to tolerate pain. But, of course, if you now live co-dependently, you are already in pain, and, chances are, your life seems out of control and tumultuous anyway. Recovery offers relief from your torment and a comforting and wonderful internal peace.

Most common definitions of recovery cite stages in the process. For example, Ernie Larsen, a pioneer in the chemical dependency field, states that:

> "1. An evolution in the process of recovery has occurred.

2. Stage I recovery is breaking the primary addiction.
3. It is vitally important to define recovery for ourselves so that we will know
   • what the real issue is
   • what to do about it
   • how to work a program to achieve that goal.
4. From the standpoint of . . . (recovery) . . . there is no difference between chemically and co-dependent persons; both must deal with underlying living problems that limit their ability to function in healthy relationships."

So recovery involves both addictive and compulsive behavior and the problems in living which cause them. John Bradshaw in *Bradshaw On: The Family* also discusses recovery in stages. Stage I recovery occurs when we recover our disabled will, that is, when we let go of our attempts to control the issues in our lives we've been trying to control. He states,

"For me the disease (co-dependence) had to wait until I dealt with its cover-up — my alcoholism. This point is crucial. For any acting-out substance abuser, the substance has to be stopped before one can treat the co-dependence (the disease of the disease). Alcoholism is caused by drinking alcohol. Alcoholism is a primary disease. This means it has to be treated first. The same is true for other drugs and chemicals.

"Food, sex, work and people addictions are somewhat different. You can't stop eating, drinking, sexing, working or peopling completely. Total abstinence would be death to self and the species. Each addiction has its own particular nuances for recovery but there are some commonalities. One commonality is surrendering the grandiose will . . .

"Stage I recovery deals with the outer layers. The outer layer defenses comprise our self-indulging habits and pain killers (our addictions) and our characterological defenses against shame. Stage I deals with our compulsive/addictive behaviors and our control madness."

Stage I helps us to re-experience our early feelings, Stage II provides a corrective experience in which we give up our old roles and scripts, and separate from our families. In Stage II we begin to forgive ourselves and our parents. Stage III takes us on a journey within to our necessary spiritual awakening.

Wayne Kritsberg in *The Adult Children of Alcoholics Syndrome* also describes recovery as a three-stage process. He discusses emotional discharge, in which we express our feelings, cognitive restructuring, which is "learning how to think in a way that is healthy and acquiring a base of information about life." And, finally, he tells us that "behavioral action" is necessary in recovery. That is when we are ". . . beginning to behave in a way that promotes a healthy lifestyle . . . beginning to take care of ourselves . . . beginning to surround ourselves with people who are themselves somewhere in the recovery process."

Exactly which issues are vital to address in recovery depends upon you as a person and upon which issues trouble you both separately and within your relationship. Some areas are troublesome to virtually all co-dependent people. These include shame, denial and dissociation from feelings, control, black-and-white thinking and negativity.

Recovery from shame begins with sharing the problems you are having. Inherent in this process is the notion that others will accept and affirm you in spite of how you see yourself or what you feel ashamed of. This process best begins in a 12-step group and in therapy where people who understand and will not condemn you are available. Shame, of course, is a major destructive element in all co-dependency and must be dealt with consistently and over time.

Part of the process of sharing your problems will involve an interruption in the denial process which accompanies your co-dependency. After years of practice, you will find that you automatically shut certain input out of consciousness. In the past this has been a survival technique, but it has also served to continue your dysfunctional and locked-in behaviors. Your denial will unravel slowly with courage and the support of the other people in your life. As your denial breaks down, you will be able to effectively handle the issues in your life in a constructive and healthy manner. While denial is firmly in place, healthy work is impossible because you are operating on only a fraction of the necessary information. Hand in hand with denial is the phenomenon of dissociation. That is, removing yourself from your feelings. As denial becomes less necessary and as you begin to develop loving and trustworthy support systems, you will learn (again, gradually) how to be comfortable with your feelings and then how to acknowledge and express them.

Control is another universal issue in the recovery from co-dependency. Most of us have spent our lives trying to control everything around us and other people, too. This is a reflection of how out of control we feel inside and our need to be perfect. Once we learn that others will accept and love us for who we are, the need to be perfect grows less urgent. We now need to face a central paradox in the recovery process: in order to be in control of ourselves in a real sense, we must surrender our will to our Higher Power. There's just too much that we, as humans, cannot influence. Compulsive behaviors are examples of this. The more we try to control them, the more out of control they feel. Here's where we need a connection to spirituality, a surrender of our will. Co-dependency, like addiction, is a spiritual disease and to heal both individually and in a relationship we require a spiritual orientation.

Black-and-white thinking and negativity are thought patterns to which co-dependents often fall victim. We also tend to reinforce such thinking within our relationships by helping each other think in these ways. Both black-and-white thinking and negativity come from and simultaneously reinforce the depression so common in co-dependency.

To change your thinking, you must first become aware of it. Try to be conscious of your automatic thoughts, even write them down. Then when you have isolated them, you can combat them by telling yourself to "Be Quiet" when you think them. You can help your spouse with this process, too. John Bradshaw's *Healing The Shame That Binds You* (Health Communications) and a workbook called *Thoughts and Feelings* (Harbinger Press) can help you further if you have a particular problem in this area.

Sometimes recovery doesn't even seem to be happening. We hit plateaus and need time to assimilate our gains. These needs must be treated with respect as, again, no one has an entirely smooth and consistent road to travel.

Self-Esteem

If you are co-dependent, almost by definition you have poor self-esteem. Recovery requires that this be corrected and that you begin to love yourself and take loving care of you. One way to enhance your self-esteem is to *"act as if"*, that is, to treat yourself as you would a much loved and appreciated friend . . . "as if" you already loved yourself. Take yourself places, surprise yourself with presents and enjoyable activities, and begin talking to yourself positively. You might also use the workbook *Thoughts and Feelings* and *Healing The Shame That Binds You* as a way to combat your negative messages to yourself.

Your relationships must be structured to support, not tear you down. Don't let others fill you with negative and self-effacing thoughts and don't let them treat you badly. Learn to say "No" or "I don't like that" by taking an assertiveness training class at your local community college.

Relationship Recovery

As you have no doubt learned, the cornerstone of a healthy relationship is a healthy individual. If you are not functional individually, you cannot function well as a couple. But each type of co-dependent relationship has special central issues which must be addressed for recovery to take place.

In every co-dependent relationship, the issue of boundaries must be resolved. Each partner needs to take individual responsibility for his or her own growth and recovery. This will delineate important boundaries between individuals.

In abuser/victim relationships, safety must be the first consideration. If physical abuse is on-going, the couple must separate and each enter individual treatment. Couple work, when it is safe to begin, should focus on power and control within the pair.

Silent type/loudmouth relationships, doctor/patient relationships, triangles, merger and arm's length relationships all have difficulty with intimacy as a central issue. If you are a part of one of these relationships, your therapy and personal growth program should contain information and process about trust and sharing and about communications.

Addictive relationships or those with compulsive behavior in evidence must be treated first by abstinence from alcohol or drugs and by modification of eating, sex, exercise, etc. Then again each individual must take responsibility for his own behavior. The enabler must focus on herself, the addict on himself.

Couple recovery depends on two healthy individuals who make the commitment to function well on their own and who want to establish intimacy between themselves. It depends on love and trust and the commitment to honesty. And it depends on separate people who are whole both within a relationship and by themselves.

When I asked Barbara and John, the successful older couple, for advice for those couples who are struggling in their marriages, they focused immediately (with no prompting from me) on the issue of boundaries.

"Even though we're very close, we're still our own people," Barbara said. "John wants me to be the best I can be, not a weakling. And we have our own interests and do our own things."

Life has not gone smoothly for John and Barbara since this writing began. Barbara has had to have surgery for cancer, and she is still receiving chemotherapy which depletes her customary energy. She is quick to express her intermittent feelings of discouragement and anger, but also tells me things could be a lot worse. John, of course, has been very concerned about her but he tries to stay positive, too.

"Even if I feel sorry for Barbara," he said, "I don't show it. I'll cry with her and support her, try to be loving, but I won't help her feel sorry for herself."

This is a good example of how people can be empathetic without being negative. This dialogue about Barbara's current problems conveys distinct and clear personal boundaries and flowing, eternal love. In addition to boundaries, Barbara and John talked extensively about forgiveness.

Both described the marital relationship as a continuous process of forgiveness.

John said, "You see both good and weakness in your partner as time goes on. Try to overlook the weakness and help if you can. What good does it do to harp on it?"

Barbara continued, "Forgiveness is really working on your own happiness. If you're married and always mad, what kind of marriage can you have? Try not to stay angry, not to punish each other, for if you hold onto anger, you stop your love and fun and growth. Without forgiveness there is no growth. You must forgive to be happy . . ."

Divorce

Sometimes marriages really are unworkable. If there is unrelenting abuse, continuous dishonesty, no feelings of love or chronic substance abuse, a couple might be forced to divorce to be self-loving. If things are very much worse than they are better or if you are the only person working on the relationship, divorce is a possibility.

John and Barbara made the point that a mistake is one thing but continuous repetition of destructive behaviors is another.

"You should concentrate on the good and work on the bad. If one person refuses to work on it or there's no improvement (on major destructive patterns) over time, divorce might be the only answer."

Of course, divorce shouldn't be taken lightly. It is a very painful and difficult decision. But a stagnant, destructive, loveless marriage shouldn't be endured forever either. Therapy can help you make a decision if you are considering divorce.

Personal Growth

Virtually everyone working in the chemical dependency field (out of which the concept of co-dependency has grown) agrees that for recovery to take place, a program of personal growth must be implemented. Larsen in *Stage II Relationships* provides some general rules which begin with a "stop and start" list to explore the habits you need to stop and those which you need to start. He continues his recommendations with the following:

Share. You need to learn to share who you are. If you want a relationship with a healthy person, that person will want to know who you are, will want to share himself or herself with you and will want you to do the same.

Stick with winners. Define who a "winner" is for you. You might decide that winners are people who are honest, who share themselves with others, who feel positive about life and living, who are happy and who enjoy life without being irresponsible. Doesn't it say a lot about you if you don't know any people like that? Find some winners — there are plenty of them around — and then stick with them.

Celebrate. That doesn't mean party all the time. It means to affirm yourself in your heart. Pat yourself on the back when you accomplish something new, however small you may think it is. Affirm yourself, celebrate your small victories over your self-defeating habits.

Have fun. Even if you are broke, there are lots of free places to go to give yourself a change of scenery.

Take care of yourself physically. Start a regular program of exercise. Improve your diet. If you are junked up on caffeine, sugar and fast foods, you are depleting the energy your body needs to fight the war against the habits you have practiced for years.

Pray. Prayer starts where your power ends.

Meditate. Meditating is being quiet enough so you can listen. Meditation is slowing yourself down so you can listen to what's inside of you.

Be financially responsible. Poor financial management really puts pressure on people. Perhaps you need to start budgeting or saving or spending. Work this out as it applies directly to you — what do you need to do to be more financially responsible?

A big part of your personal growth program should be a 12-step group. The 12 steps will help you come to terms with your shame and with your control issues. If you abuse substances, sex, food or gambling, there are specific 12-step or "anonymous" programs for you. If your issues are about your dysfunctional family, you need to look into either an Adult Children of Alcoholics group through Al-Anon (you don't have to be from an alcoholic family; any dysfunctional family will do) or a Co-dependents Anonymous group (CODA). These groups can be located by calling the service centers for each, phone numbers for which are usually located in your local telephone directory. If you have trouble finding their number, I suggest you call a local alcoholism treatment center for the Al-Anon service center. They will probably be able to provide you with information regarding the other groups as well. (See Appendix for addresses.) In addition to helping you grapple with issues, a group will give you a support system to help you on your journey.

You will want to read everything you can get your
hands on regarding the dysfunctional family and co-
dependency, and you will want to share the literature
with your spouse. (See Suggested Reading list.) It is
always helpful to learn everything you can about
yourself, your marriage and your family of origin.

Therapy

Find a therapist who is willing to do both individual
and couples therapy. His or her discipline doesn't matter.
The emotional connection you are able to establish does.
As long as the person is a professionally trained
therapist with whom you can feel close, you will be able
to work together. Although some vocabulary will be
different, your therapist should have a working knowledge of most of the following:

1. Family systems theory and the systems nature of
   family disturbances. This is the concept which
   explains how interconnected we are with our
   families; that when one member grows and
   changes, so do the other members.
2. Some knowledge of substance abuse and compulsive behavior
3. An awareness of shame and how it affects people
4. An understanding of the dysfunctional family
   and co-dependency.

The Process

There is no time limit for the process of recovery.
Most of us will be involved in one way or another for
our entire lives. Your support systems should help you
grow, both as individuals and as a couple. After some of
your individual issues are resolved, couples therapy will
be a place to learn how to communicate and how to stay
out of your predictable conflicts.

Recovery takes a lifetime. The journey required to be all that you can be, whole and alive, is a long one. I am reminded of sitting with my husband and watching John Bradshaw's public television series *"On The Family"*. We had watched about half of the ten episodes. During the sixth, I turned to look at Larry and was startled to find him sitting with his head in his hands looking distressed and forlorn.

"What's the matter?" I asked him. I was very concerned.

"When can we stop growing?" he asked, looking sad, but with a twinkle in his eye.

"Never, I hope . . ."

Larry was teasing me, but I was serious. If growth stops, so does meaningful life.

You have seen the faces of the co-dependent marriage, how it happens and what to do about it. You have also had a short glimpse into a healthy marriage. I hope that *In Sickness and in Health* will help you through your path toward personal and relationship transformation.

SUGGESTED READING

Ables and Brandsma, *Therapy for Couples* (Jossey-Bass), 1977.

Ackerman, Robert, *Let Go and Grow* (Health Communications), 1987.

Bowlby, John, *The Making and Breaking of Affectional Bonds* (Tavistock), 1979.

Beavers, W., *Successful Marriage* (WW Norton), 1985. *Psychotherapy and Growth* (Brunner-Mazel), 1977.

Black, Claudia, *It Will Never Happen to Me* (MAC), 1982.

Bradshaw, John, *Bradshaw On: The Family*, 1987. *Healing The Shame That Binds You* (Health Communications), 1988.

Carnes, Patrick, *Out of the Shadows* (CompCare), 1983.

Erikson, E., *Childhood and Society* (WW Norton), 1950.

Fossum, M. and Mason, M., *Facing Shame* (WW Norton), 1986.

Friel and Friel, *Adult Children* (Health Communications), 1988.

Gravitz and Bowden, *Recovery: A Guide for Adult Children of Alcoholics* (Simon and Schuster), 1987.

Guerin, Fay, Burden and Kautto, *The Evaluation and Treatment of Marital Conflict* (Basic Books), 1987.

Hafner, R. Julian, *Marriage and Mental Illness* (Guilford), 1986.

Kaplan, Helen Singer, *Disorders of Sexual Desire* (Brunner-Mazel), 1979.

Kritsberg, Wayne, *The ACoA Syndrome* (Health Communications), 1985.

Larsen, Ernie, *Stage II Recovery*, 1985. *Stage II Relationships* (Harper and Row), 1987.

Miller, Alice, *Prisoners of Childhood* (Basic Books), 1981.

NiCarthy, Ginny, *Getting Free* (Seal Press), 1982.

Norwood, Robin, *Women Who Love Too Much* (Pocket Books), 1985.

Peck, M. Scott, *The Road Less Traveled* (Simon and Schuster), 1978.

Peele, Stanton, *Love and Addiction* (Signet), 1975.

Satir, Virginia, *Peoplemaking*, 1972. *Conjoint Family Therapy*, (Science and Behavior Books), 1964.

Scarf, Maggie, *Intimate Partners*, (Random House), 1987.

Schaef, Anne, *Co-Dependence*, 1986. *When Society Becomes an Addict* (Harper and Row), 1987.

Schaeffer, Brenda, *Is It Love Or Is It Addiction?* (Hazelden), 1987.

Siexas and Youch, *Children of Alcoholism* (Harper and Row), 1985.

Stahmann and Herbert, *Klermer's Counseling in Marital and Sexual Problems* (Williams and Wilkins), 1977.

Stuart and Orr, *Otherwise Perfect* (Health Communications), 1987.

Subby, Robert, *Lost in the Shuffle* (Health Communications), 1987.

Walker, Lenore, *The Battered Woman* (Harper and Row), 1979.

Whitfield, Charles, *Healing the Child Within* (Health Communications), 1987.

Willi, Jurg, *Couples in Collusion* (Hunter House), 1975.

Woititz, Janet, *Adult Children of Alcoholics*, 1983. *Marriage on the Rocks*, 1979. *Struggle for Intimacy* (Health Communications), 1985.

APPENDIX

- Al-Anon, Al-Anon Adult
  Children of Alcoholics and
  Alateen Family Groups
  POB 862 Midtown Station
  New York, NY 10018
- Alcoholics Anonymous
  Box 459 Grand Central
  Station
  New York, NY 10163
- Adult Children of Alcoholics
  POB 35623
  Los Angeles, CA 90035
- Batterers Anonymous
  POB 29
  Redlands, CA 92373
- Co-dependents
  Anonymous
  POB 5508
  Glendale, AZ 85312-5508
  (602) 944-0141
- Divorce Anonymous
  POB 5313
  Chicago, IL 60680

- Emotions Anonymous
  POB 4245
  St. Paul, MN 55104
- Families Anonymous
  POB 344
  Torrance, CA 90501
- Families in Action
  Suite 300
  3845 N. Druid Hills Rd.
  Decatur, GA 30033
- Incest Survivors
  Anonymous
  POB 5613
  Long Beach, CA 90805
- Nar-Anon Family Groups
  350 5th St., Suite 207
  San Pedro, CA 90731
- Narcotics Anonymous
  POB 9999
  Van Nuys, CA 91409
- National Single Parent
  Coalition
  10 West 23 Street
  New York, NY 10010

- Overeaters Anonymous
  4025 Spenser St.,
  Suite 203
  Torrance, CA 90503
- Parents Anonymous
  22330 Hawthorne Blvd.
  Torrance, CA 90505
- Parents Without Partners
  7910 Woodmont Ave.
  Washington, DC 20014
- Pill-Anon Family
  Programs
  POB 120 Gracie Station
  New York, NY 10028

- Pills Anonymous
  POB 473 Ansonia
  Station
  New York, NY 10023

- Prison Families
  Anonymous
  134 Jackson Street
  Hempstead, NY 11550

- Single Dad's Hotline
  POB 4842
  Scottsdale, AZ 85258

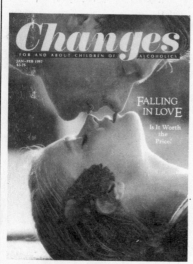